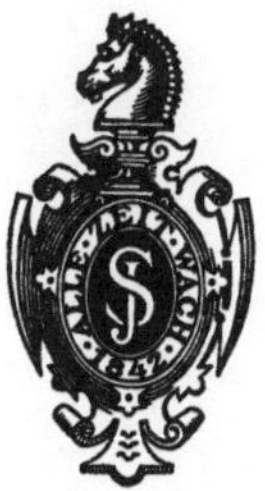

A. Wackenheim · J. P. Braun

Angiography of the Mesencephalon

Normal and Pathological Findings

With 128 Figures

Springer-Verlag Berlin Heidelberg GmbH 1970

Prof. agr. A. Wackenheim, Head of the Neuroradiological Department
C. H. U. de Strasbourg, France

Dr. J. P. Braun, Head of the Neuroradiological Department C. H. R. Colmar,
France

ISBN 978-3-662-27882-6   ISBN 978-3-662-29384-3 (eBook)
DOI 10.1007/978-3-662-29384-3

Preface

In the beginning after Dandy's publication in 1918, ventriculography and pneumencephalography were the main tools in the neuroradiographical examination of brain tumours.

Later on, cerebral angiography after Egaz Moniz in 1927, has been more and more commonly used. Now it appears to be the most important neuroradiological examination in tumours of the great hemispheres.

Up till some years ago, air studies were the predominant examinations in lesions of the brainstem and the contents of the posterior fossa. Gradually angiographic examination for lesions in these regions has been more frequently used.

Nowadays angiographic examination of the mesencephalon proves to be of increasing importance. However, some neuroradiologists feel inhibited. They fear difficulties when reading the angiogram, even if the subtraction method is applied.

Like other workers in the field of neuroradiology and neurosurgery they will be very pleased with the edition of Wackenheim and Braun's monograph.

These authors are already well known because of their excellent air studies in mesencephalic lesions. With this book they provide us with a most valuable and clear guide to the interpretation of normal and pathologic angiograms, including capillarograms, of the mesencephalic regions.

August 6th, 1970   B. G. Ziedses des Plantes

Acknowledgments

This treatise is the result of a paper presented in Cologne in 1968 on tumours of the posterior region of the IIIrd ventricle. Our thanks go to Professor K. Zülch for the confidence he was good enough to have in our work by asking us to handle this subject at that time.

Our thanks are due also to Professor C. Gros, Professor F. Rohmer, Professor D. Phillippidès, Professor E. Woringer and Doctor J. Baumgartner whose wide experience in the pathology of the nervous system was of great help to us.

We address our thanks equally to Dean F. Isch who was good enough to favor the creation of the European Society of Neuroradiology in Colmar by participating actively in the colloquium consecrated to the nervous system of the posterior fossa.

A special acknowledgment goes to Doctor N. Heldt for her highly competent anatomic dissections.

Acknowledgments are in order to Professor Y. Legal who was obliging enough to welcome us at the Institute of Pathological Anatomy in Strasbourg, and to Doctor A. Tänzer of Hamburg who was kind enough to pass on to us certain radiographic documents.

We thank also our technical assistants in Colmar and Strasbourg who handled the work of subtraction and medical photography, and Mrs. L. Braun for her English translation of our text.

Finally our thanks go to two great masters of Neuroradiology, Professor B. Ziedses des Plantes and Doctor James Bull whose support in the founding of the European Society of Neuroradiology makes possible that our monograph appear as the first work published by members of the Society as such. May they find here the expression of our admiration and respect.

Auguste Wackenheim, M.D.   Jean-Paul Braun, M.D.
Strasbourg   Colmar

January 17, 1970

Contents

Contents

Introduction

The vascularisation of the mesencephalon differs from that of other regions of the brain in that it presents more difficulties, so much so that mesencephalic angiography is not reputed to be sure. We shall see that a wider knowledge of the arteries and veins of this region diminishes considerably these misgivings.

The mesencephalic arteries are relatively thin. Their morphological analysis demands not only well contrasted and sharp radiographs but also complementary procedures to improve the picture's quality and whose application requires a real "laboratory of the radiographic picture". Among the different radiographic methods, Ziedses Des Plantes' subtraction takes the lead. We shall see in this paper that it is absolutely indispensable to the study of the mesencephalic region.

While normal angiographic analysis is relatively easy in lateral views, it is much more difficult in frontal views. Efforts to better the picture produce only mediocre results in frontal views of the normal mesencephalic arteries. Often the superimposition of the superior cerebellar arteries overshadows these views. Under certain pathological conditions the mesencephalic arteries are sufficiently enlarged so as to be clearly distinguishable from the superior cerebellar arteries. However, small avascular tumors present difficulties of interpretation; they appear as negative capillarographic views, that is, as avascular areas (Fig. 83). Vertebral angiographies in a Towne or axial view are of little help. Nevertheless, we shall see that this aspect is of some value in analyzing certain deformations in the peripeduncular loop of the posterior cerebral artery.

Problems in angiography differ basically depending on whether one seeks criteria of normality or whether one wishes to diagnose visible anomalies. Since one turns to ischemic pathology in the search for criteria of normality the results are disappointing. On the other hand, when one is confronted with arterial anomalies, things are much easier. An analysis of shiftings and deformations leads to an accurate topographic diagnosis and sometimes even to an indication as to the cause. We shall not work out any further this idea but shall simply recall to mind those facile aspects provided by spontaneously opacified lesions such as congenital vascular malformations, glioblastomas, teratomas, meningiomas and ependymomas.

Another difficulty is of a clinical nature: a mesencephalic syndrome is rarely typical, so much so that the angiographic application can vary from the carotidal to the vertebral field. Carotido-vertebral angiographies do not solve the problem of the mesencephalon. The thinness of mesencephalic arteries demands a high degree of selectivity. The choice between carotidal and vertebral angiography is more difficult in that the carotid furnishes an incomplete view of the posterior cerebral artery since the initial segment remains unseen. Since the medial posterior choroidal artery arises from this segment, it is always necessary to make an angiographic study of the mesencephalon by vertebral means.

The mesencephalon is a virtual crossroads in hydrocephaly, and angiographic diagnosis is of the utmost importance in this syndrome. Therefore, we shall attempt to evaluate mesencephalic angiography along these lines.

The mesencephalic veins are more easily identified than the arteries. They are of a higher calibre and are made up of such invariable elements such as Galen's vein, Rosenthal's basal vein and others, such as the thalamic veins, the lateral and posterior mesencephalic veins, the interpeduncular veins and the anterior pontomesencephalic veins. The method of subtraction permits the realization of excellent pictures whose interpretation is less hazardous than it was.

We shall try to deal with the problems of normal and pathological capillarography. In our opinion, this technique has a future. While we cannot see the capillary vessels of the brain, we can at the present time follow the contrast fluid in these vessels through the spread stain. This procedure is possible only in a department where subtraction is used. Moreover, in the topographic sense, the arterial network complements the venous one. Figs. 2 and 5 demonstrate this well. The veins of the vertebrobasilar system are found in the medial antero-superior mesencephalic and lateral inferior regions. The arteries, on the other hand, are found in the medial and lateral superior mesencephalon. The topographic dissociation of the mesencephalic arteries and veins can but increase the interest we have in phlebographic study.

The mesencephalon is reputed to be of little neurosurgical interest. Neuroradiological investigation has suffered from this underevaluation. We shall see how this region is suited to certain surgery since extracerebral tumours often react as intracerebral ones from the neurological point of view. An angiographic study permits to differentiate the two forms.

On numerous occasions medial sagittal pneumostratigraphy has furnished us the means with which to diagnose tumours of the mesencephalon. We have been advocating it since 1958 as routine procedure in gas encephalography. Fig. 1 gives examples of pictures taken with this technique. They do not define the nature of the tumour, and in any case the vascularisation of mesencephalic tumours must be studied by means of vertebral angiography. Moreover, capillarography discloses tumoral opacifications which we shall call "positive", while normal capillary stains make it possible to establish the limits of avascular pinealomas by producing "negative" areas. Unfortunately not all cases yield these types of views. In the final analysis the attending physician or surgeon is the sole judge as to the application of this angiographic technique. Mesencephalic angiography, as we shall demonstrate in this paper, deserves a better place than it has.

In the mesencephalon, as elsewhere, special cases may come up which serve to round out and confirm the neuroradiology of this region (Figs. 3 and 4). Our paper does not concentrate on these but rather will try to present as clearly as possible our general experience of three years' standing in this field.

Review of Literature

Works concerned with the mesencephalon are relatively few in number. Reference will be made to those publications we have consulted. We have doubtlessly overlooked some works and we beg the authors here and now to excuse these inevitable omissions.

The *arteries* have been submitted to detailed anatomical and radioanatomical analysis and we shall have little to add to previous descriptions. Our emphasis will be placed on pathological arteriograms.

The *veins* of the mesencephalon have been the object of less detailed study. This is understandable when one considers that the arterial system involves difficulties of interpretation and that the veins present a large anatomical variety as well as differences in time of opacification. There are many papers concerned with the deep phlebogram, but there is a definite lack of works dealing with the mesencephalic veins. We have been led to attempt, therefore, a supplement to current knowledge of the normal and pathologic mesencephalic phlebogram.

A. Papers on the Arteries

Considerable confusion reigns in the nomenclature of the arteries of the mesencephalic area. In our study we shall summarize the principal works concerned with this subject. Furthermore, we can state as of now that the study of approximately 1,000 vertebral angiograms permits us to classify *three groups* of arteries, front to back:

1. The posterior thalamo-perforating arteries (arteriae thalamoperforatae posteriores).
2. The colliculi quadrigemini and corpori geniculati arteries (arteriae colliculi quadrigemini et corpori geniculati).
3. The posterior choroidal arteries (arteriae chorioideae posteriores).

This classification is purely angiographic. Reference to anatomic works reveals a higher degree of complexity in the arterial system of the mesencephalon. This complexity is real and has been substantiated by dissection. In mesencephalic angiography, only the above-mentioned groups are visible in lateral projections. The identification of these arteries is more difficult in fronto-suboccipital projections. It is almost impossible in axial and half-axial projections in spite of the use, under the best possible conditions, of subtraction. In pathological cases, however, these arteries are visible in frontal projections.

H. Rouvière's Works (1940)

In his work on human anatomy, Rouvière distinguishes the following arteries:
—*the arteries of the cerebral peduncles* which arise from the basilar artery and from the posterior cerebral arteries. They extend as far as the peri-aqueducal grey matter. These arteries correspond to our "group of posterior thalamo-perforating arteries".
—*the anterior and middle arteries of the colliculi quadrigemini* arise from the posterior cerebral artery and vascularise the posterior quadrigeminal bodies. These arteries are included in the second group, the "colliculi quadrigemini and corpori geniculati arteries".
—*the posterior arteries of the colliculi quadrigemini*, according to Rouvière, arise from the superior cerebellar arteries in order to vascularise the posterior segment of the posterior quadrigeminal bodies, the superior cerebellar peduncles and the antero-superior wall of the IVth ventricle. We have never seen a picture corresponding to such arteries.

P. Namin's Works (1955)

Namin distinguishes:
the peduncular arteries
the optic arteries
the posterior choroidal arteries
the quadrigeminal arteries

1. Peduncular Arteries

Internal Arteries : these small arteries arise from the extremity of the basilar trunk. They also issue from the first segment of the posterior cerebral artery and from the posterior communicating artery. They are terminal and irrigate the tegmentum, the lemniscus medialis, the nucleus ruber, the superior cerebellar peduncle, and the nuclei of the IIIrd and IVth cranial nerves.
External Arteries : they have the same origins as the internal branches but can also originate from the superior cerebellar

artery and the anterior choroidal artery. They irrigate the external part of the tegmentum.

2. Optic Arteries

These are branches of the posterior cerebral artery. We believe that they may also arise from the posterior choroidal arteries. Since their angiographic individualization seems problematical, we shall not take these arteries into account. Namin describes the inferior optic arteries which supply the lateral wall of the IIIrd ventricle and the internal side of the thalamus. He also describes the posterior and internal optic arteries which supply the postero-internal side of the thalamus. Finally, he reports the presence of the posterior and external optic arteries relegated to the postero-external side of the thalamus.

3. The Posterior Choroidal Arteries

a) Posterior and Lateral Choroidal Artery

This artery arises from the posterior cerebral artery behind the peduncle and divides into two branches:
an external branch intended for the superior part of the choroidal plexus of the lateral ventricle.
an internal branch for the tela chorioidea of the IIIrd ventricle.

b) Posterior Middle Choroidal Artery

One branch supplies the pineal gland while the other two are terminal arteries:
—an internal one for the tela chorioidea,
—an external one for the choroidal plexus of the lateral ventricle.

4. Arteries of the Corpori Quadrigemini

Namin describes three arteries which issue from the posterior cerebral artery: one for the anterior quadrigeminal bodies, another for the posterior corpus and a third artery for the intercorporeal area.

The Works of Columella (1956)

The author lays stress on the semeiology of the posterior cerebral artery which permits to localise pineal tumours and such extra-cerebral tumours in this area as meningiomas of the free edge of the tentorium. The internal occipital artery is lifted by meningiomas and lowered by pinealomas. We wish to render hommage to Columella who undertook the study of these types of tumours well before us.

The Works of Lazorthes and his Coworkers (1956—1961)

In their study concerned with cerebral vascularisation, the authors enumerate the central cortical branches of the posterior cerebral artery.

The central or meso-diencephalic branches are divided into four groups. These arteries originate in the proximal segment of the posterior cerebral artery (precommunicating segment). In 1968 Professor Lazorthes confirmed the data reported hereinafter.

1. The Interpeduncular Arteries

(Foix and Hillemand's retromammillary pedicle) Lazorthes and his coworkers describe:

—*an anterior or diencephalic group*, situated in front of and at the level of the mammillary tubercles. It includes arteries which supply the hypothalamus and the ventral nuclei of the thalamus.

—*a posterior or mesencephalic group*, situated behind the mammillary tubercles. This group is found in the interpeduncular cistern and vascularises the cerebral peduncle, the nucleus ruber, the locus niger, the sub-thalamic area and the superior cerebellar peduncle.

2. The Quadrigeminal Arteries

These arise from the posterior cerebral artery ahead of the posterior communicating artery (precommunicating segment.) Two branches may be distinguished, one for the anterior quadrigeminal body, and the other for the posterior one.

3. The Posterior Choroidal Arteries

—Lazorthes holds that the posterior choroidal arteries may have an isolated origin or issue from a common trunk.

—*The main or medial posterior choroidal artery* passes around the cerebral peduncle spreading six or seven branches which vascularise the anterior quadrigeminal tubercles as well. The first two segments are concave forward, the second of which runs along the lateral margin of the pineal gland parallel to the great vein of Galen and ending in several branches in the tela chorioidea and in the superior choroidal plexus.

—*The accessory or lateral posterior choroidal artery* runs along the supero-internal margin of the thalamus, vascularises the internal part of the body of the nucleus caudatus and anastomises with the anterior choroidal artery.

4. Lazorthes' Posterior and Lateral Thalamic Arteries

(Foix and Hillemand's thalamo-geniculate pedicle or Duret's infero-external optic artery).

These arteries penetrate into the internal part of the external geniculate body and vascularise the postero-lateral part of the thalamus, the posterior part of the internal capsule and the external part of Wernicke's area.

Given our angiographic data, we believe that the aforementioned systematization can be found, in part, in arteriograms along the following lines:

—*arteriae thalamo-perforatae posteriores*. These correspond to Lazorthes' posterior interpeduncular arteries and to Foix and Hillemand's peduncular arteries.

—*arteriae colliculi quadrigemini et corpori geniculati*. These correspond to Lazorthes' quadrigeminal arteries, to his posterior and lateral thalamic arteries, to Foix and Hillemand's thalamo-geniculate pedicle or to Duret's infero-external optic artery.

—*arteriae chorioideae posteriores*. Everyone agrees with this designation. The size of these arteries is important enough to permit us to recognize them rather clearly in angiograms.

F. O. Löfgren's Works (1958)

Löfgren's study ranks among the most important works. It concerns solely the diagnosis of pineal tumours, to the exclusion of other tumours of the mesencephalic area. We wish to remind our readers that it was Radner's method that was first used in vertebral angiography. This author was a forerunner in this field. At present the retrograde angiographic method is generally employed via the brachial, axillary and femoral arteries.

Löfgren shows very schematically the anatomy of the posterior choroidal arteries. As we shall see later, his diagram will be criticized by Galloway. According to Löfgren:

The *medial posterior choroidal artery* supplies the choroidal plexus of the IIIrd ventricle. It issues from the cerebral artery and runs along the lateral margin of the pineal gland towards the tela chorioidea of the IIIrd ventricle following the course of the internal cerebral vein.

The *lateral posterior choroidal artery* also issues from the posterior cerebral artery and runs parallel with it in a short course before going around the thalamus and ending in the choroidal plexus of the lateral ventricle. This artery is designated as "main branch" by Löfgren who worked out measurements from 100 lateral vertebral angiograms. These measurements are still valid today.

Löfgren's first guidemark is established by the distance between the extremity of the basal trunk and the most posterior point of the artery. This distance is plotted on a straight line which runs parallel to the direction of the posterior cerebral artery. Normally this distance measures 30 to 45 mm.

Löfgren's second guidemark is taken from the largest distance which separates the extremity of the basilar artery from the lateral posterior choroidal artery. This distance measures, as does the first one, about 30 to 45 mm, with an average of 35 to 40 mm.

Löfgren's third guidemark is based on the distance between the extremity of the basilar artery and the extremity of the lateral posterior choroidal artery. It measures 25 to 40 mm. Because of the variability in terminal filling of these small arteries, we feel that this third point is of lesser importance.

We shall see that Löfgren's measurements are of real general interest. They serve in teaching, in settling differences of opinion or in dispelling doubt. Aware of the relative value of these measurements, we have drawn up a slightly modified diagram to be used in iconography. Such a diagram has the advantage of helping the radiologist to commit to memory the area of normal lateral projection of the posterior choroidal arteries.

In cases of tumours in the pineal region, Löfgren indicates a symmetrical displacement upwards and backwards of the posterior choroidal arteries effecting an unwinding curve. These modifications were found in 10 out of 21 cases of pineal tumours. Löfgren further indicates that in 3 of these 10 cases the displacement was solely upwards of the posterolateral choroidal artery. There was no displacement backwards.

Löfgren recalls that hydrocephaly can cause rigidity of the posterior cerebral artery. He points out that posterior thalamic tumours can cause the same arterial deformation as pineal tumours, but that these deformations are asymmetrical or unilateral (3 cases out of 6). In three other cases of posterior thalamic tumours, the author observed an opposite displacement of the posterior choroidal arteries, that is frontwards and downwards. However, the only picture he gives is not convincing. As to the frontal image of these arteries, Löfgren does not deal with the question, insisting upon the difficulties of identification. He does point out, however, that the lateral expansion of a pineal tumour is found in one case by a medial displacement of the anterior cerebral artery, and in another by an opposite displacement of the superior cerebellar artery.

As for the venous system, Löfgren's works are academical, based on the internal cerebral veins, the basal veins and the great vein of Galen. Let us note, however, that he points out the existence of visible thalamic veins under the internal cerebral vein. Tumours of the pineal region displace the internal cerebral vein upwards and backwards. The usual normal S-shaped configuration of the vein of Galen and the cerebral vein is broken and angular. Löfgren feels that venous deformations of this nature are more precocious than deformations of the posterior choroidal arteries in pineal tumours and that the contrary is true in cases of thalamic tumours.

In conclusion, Löfgren tries to establish a correlation between angiographic anomalies and the size of a pineal tumour:

—a tumour measuring 2.5×3 cm or more can cause arterial and venous displacements;

—a tumour measuring 2.5×2.5 cm or less causes no displacement, but can modify the internal cerebral vein;

—a tumour measuring 2.5×2 cm modifies neither the arteries nor the veins.

We shall see that such tumours can be identified by capillarography.

C. Thevenot's Works (1959)

The author enumerates the following tributaries of the posterior cerebral artery:

—interpeduncular arteries which arise from the bifurcation of the basilar trunk and spread in the optostriate region;

—external peduncular arteries in the opto-peduncular sulcus;

—middle arteries of the quadrigeminal bodies;

—arteries of the corpori geniculati;

—anterior arteries of the quadrigeminal bodies;

—arteries of the hippocampus;

—posterior thalamo-perforating arteries;

—posterior and lateral choroidal arteries;

—posterior and middle choroidal arteries.

The arteries mentioned above do not appear on the radiograms reproduced in the author's work.

E. Pernkopf's Works (1960)

According to the author, the posterior choroidal artery is formed by two arteries:

10

—a middle choroidal artery issuing from the superior cerebellar artery;

—a lateral choroidal artery which separates from the posterior cerebral artery.

K. Decker's Works (1960)

The author emphasizes the wealth of pneumographic information and the poor diagnostic yield of angiographic examinations.

The Works of R. Galloway and T. Greitz (1960)

Two years after Löfgren's studies, Galloway and Greitz publish an important paper on the posterior choroidal arteries which they call "medial and lateral choroid arteries".

a) The Middle Choroidal Artery. We designate this artery in our monograph under the latin term "arteria chorioidea posteromedialis". We feel that the designation "posterior" must be preserved in order to distinguish this artery from the "arteria chorioidea anterior". We also feel that it would be better to retain the latin terminology in order to avoid the usual confusion.

According to Galloway and Greitz, this artery arises in the initial segment of the posterior cerebral artery in the interpeduncular cistern. It runs parallel to the posterior cerebral artery, close to the cerebral trunk and emerges in Galen's cistern next to the pineal body which it supplies. In a lateral view, the artery describes a figure "3", that is to say, a double anterior concavity. The upper concavity corresponds to the merging of the artery which joins the roof of the IIIrd ventricle. At this level it vascularises the choroidal plexus of the IIIrd ventricle and sometimes supplies a small branch for the choroidal plexus of the lateral ventricle. Galloway and Löfgren disagree over a fundamental point in angiography. According to Galloway, the artery is lateral-pineal, whereas Löfgren feels it runs above the pineal gland. Under these conditions, a pinealoma obviously would involve quite different displacements depending whether the artery is situated on the posterior side or on the lateral side of the tumour.

b) Lateral Choroidal Arteries. The most important fact described by Galloway and Greitz is the existence of two lateral arteries. The anterior artery separates from the posterior cerebral artery in its latero-peduncular course and penetrates immediately the choroidal fissure to supply the plexus of the temporal horn. The size (length and calibre) of the lateroanterior artery is inversely proportional to that of the anterior choroidal artery. In general, this lateral anterior choroidal artery is much thinner than its posterior homologue. The latter also separates from the posterior cerebral artery in the lateropeduncular cistern to enter into the choroidal fissure. In its sub-thalamic course, the artery has two branches. A larger lateral branch joins the internal part of the plexus of the temporal horn on the posterior side of the trigone. The internal branch, usually thinner, winds around the thalamus in a large anterior concavity to terminate in the tela chorioidea.

According to Galloway and Greitz, there is a relationship in size between the anterior and posterior artery, the former compensating by its larger size the narrowness of the latter. When one of the two is missing the other is thicker and passes behind the thalamus outlining its posterior contour.

The work of Galloway and Greitz permits to determine normal radioanatomy. Given ideal conditions, six posterior choroidal arteries can be identified:

a left postero-medial choroidal artery
a right postero-medial choroidal artery
a left antero-lateral posterior choroidal artery
a right antero-lateral posterior choroidal artery
a left postero-lateral posterior choroidal artery
a right postero-lateral posterior choroidal artery

As a matter of fact, we have been able to identify the six arteries only in certain lateral projections, as we shall show later on. The superimposition of six vessels is rare and not well explained. It appears that only 4 posterior choroidal arteries are sufficiently large to be opacified by contrast fluid. The four arteries easily identified in lateral projections are the 2 medial choroidal and the 2 lateral choroidal arteries. At times, due to hemodynamics, the choroidal arteries are opacified on one side only.

Clinical angiography is not elaborated in Galloway's work. He feels that these arteries are not easily identifiable in frontal projections and doubts their identification in lateral projections as well. Arterial displacements observed in pathological cases are enumerated as follows by Galloway and Greitz:

—*a pineal tumour* displaces the medial artery. When the lateral choroidal artery is displaced towards the rear, the tumour occupies the thalamic area.

—*a tumour situated more to the rear,* such as a meningioma of the tentorial edge, involves a displacement of the medial choroidal artery towards the front;

—*a thalamic tumour* increases the course of the homolateral posterolateral choroidal artery.

The Works of Krayenbühl and Yasargil (1962)

These authors have well described the modifications of the deep phlebogram in the case of thalamic tumours. They insist upon the value of vertebral angiography to demonstrate the displacement of the posterior choroidal arteries or in the spontaneous opacification of mesencephalic tumours. However, the work of Krayenbühl and Yasargil adds no new element to earlier works.

The Works of Potts and Taveras (1963)

These authors summarize angiographic anomalies found in cases of thalamic tumours:

Lateral View: an elevation of the sylvian fissure and the middle cerebral arteries had been observed, as well as a downward displacement of the anterior choroidal artery sometimes outlining the posterior aspect of the enlarged thalamus, an elevation of the internal cerebral vein, and of the thalamostriate vein, with an opening of the venous angle. The authors insist on the fact that tumours of the posterior part of the IIIrd ventricle involve an elevation of the posterior segment of the internal cerebral vein and that this elevation is particularly visible when one compares the vein on the tumour side with the normal side.

Frontal View: there may be a widening of the space between the anterior cerebral artery and the middle cerebral artery; a variable displacement of the anterior choroidal and lenticulostriate arteries. The most common finding was elevation of the internal cerebral vein with displacement across the midline. The authors demonstrate that ventricular dilatation is responsible for the typically broad concave upward curve.

The Works of M. David and Cow. (1965)

Their work reassesses Foix and Hillemand's classification and adapts the notions previously exposed by Galloway and Greitz (1964) and by Lazorthes (1961).

The Works of G. Westberg (1966)

Westberg recalls the confusion in anatomic and radiologic literature in the naming of vessels in the posterior arterial system. Names such as praemammillary or thalamo-tuberal, retro-mammillary or thalamo-perforating and thalamo-geniculate arteries are commonly encountered.

Westberg proposes to name the vessel arising from the posterior communicating artery and which penetrates into the base of the brain the anterior thalamo-perforating artery. This vessel is quite visible in a lateral angiographic projection when the posterior communicating artery is opacified. Westberg shows that it penetrates the brain lateral to the mammillary body and that it supplies the antero-lateral regions of the thalamus. In consequence, this vessel does not pertain to our study.

The posterior thalamo-perforating arteries issue from the posterior cerebral artery and run into the interpeduncular fossa. These arteries correspond to those we call, as Westberg, "arteriae thalamo-perforatae posteriores" and whose morphologic peculiarities we shall point out later on.

In his work concerned with the arteries of the basal ganglia, Westberg does not take issue with the problems posed by the mesencephalic arteries as such. Finally Westberg restates some pathological findings concerning ventricular dilatation (p. 586), vascular diseases (p. 589), expanding lesions (p. 590).

The Works of North (1966)

The angiographic problem connected with mesencephalic tumours was presented in North's thesis without the addition of new facts.

The Works of Djindjian and Bories (1967)

The authors have elaborated a didactic study in which they distinguish:

—*pineal tumours* which modify primarily the postero-medial or main choroidal artery displacing it towards the front (seen laterally inversed concavity). May we remind our readers that Löfgren had already pointed out this fact. We shall also add an example (Fig. 84).

—*tumours of the posterior part of the IIIrd ventricle* which cause most especially an elevation to the level of the postero-medial choroidal artery.

—thalamic tumours modify the thalamo-perforating arteries as well as the postero-lateral choroidal arteries. The postero-medial arteries are not displaced.

—tumours of the splenium corporis callosi produce a mass expanding lesion which pushes the posterior pericallosal artery towards the back and the postero-medial choroidal artery towards the front.

The Works of Ruggiero (1967)

This author summarizes the works of Duret, Foix and Lazorthes and distinguishes:

—the interpeduncular arteries,

—the quadrigeminal arteries,

—the posterior choroidal arteries.

Ruggiero recalls that Greitz and Galloway report two lateral posterior choroidal arteries, an anterior one and a posterior one, while Lazorthes on the other hand feels there is only the postero-lateral choroidal artery, itself a terminal branch of the postero-medial choroidal artery.

A. Isfort's Works (1967)

This author enumerates the branches of the posterior cerebral artery, among others, the posterior perforating arteries, the quadrigeminal arteries, the choroidal arteries and a collateral for the splenium corporis callosi. It is rare to come across an author who reports the presence of this posterior pericallosal branch whose angiographic importance is considerable in localizing mesencephalic tumours.

The Works of Zatz and Cow. (1967)

These authors present a study of five tumours of the splenium based solely on carotid angiography. The authors insist on the importance of the displacements of the posterior pericallosal artery responsible for the spontaneous tumoural opacification found in three cases. In this work, it is recalled that the space which separates the internal cerebral vein from the inferior longitudinal sinus depends on the variable development of the falx. The posterior cerebral vein furnishes on the other hand a good indication of the level of the postero-superior edge of the corpus callosi.

The Works of Decker and Backmund (1968)

In their work concerned with cerebral circulation, the authors report a glioblastoma of the posterior part of the IIIrd ventricle. They emphasize the heavy tumoural vascularisation in the posterior choroidal area.

Personal Works

Wackenheim, Braun and Bradac (1968)

We have presented the over-all mesencephalic problem in a report submitted to the German Society of Neuroradiology in Cologne in 1968. The essential elements of this report will be given in this work. Our ideas have further evolved since the presentation of our report, which at that time we were obliged to give schematically.

B. Papers on the Veins

The cerebral venous system has been classified, sometimes in contradictory fashion, by numerous anatomists. It was first studied in neuroradiology by Johanson. In 1954 he described the course of the basal vein, certain small veins of the cerebral peduncle, the pons and the medial part of the temporal lobe. Subsequently Lindgren and cow. on the one hand, Krayenbühl, Yasargil and Richter, on the other, contributed works of equal importance. The school of Lille made contributions on the phlebogram in the persons of Laine, Delandsheer and Galibert.

The veins of the posterior fossa have been particularly well studied by Huang who based his work on embryological and anatomical observations. Huang first defined the normal radioanatomy of these veins in a paper published in 1961. In the mesencephalic region proper Huang has described the precentral vein, the lateral mesencephalic vein, the ponto-mesencephalic vein and the interpeduncular veins, as well as such drainage variants of the basal vein as the lateral anastomic mesencephalic vein, and the great anterior cerebellar vein.

Viale and Rosa (1968) studied on their own the veins of the posterior fossa and submitted quite interesting angiographic documents.

The meeting in Colmar (1969) has proved the importance of the mesencephalic venous system. We refer the reader to the reports of this meeting, to be published in "Neuroradiology" 1970.

Normal Findings

Normal Radioanatomy of the Arteries

1. Posterior Cerebral Arteries

Frontal View. The posterior cerebral artery is the terminal branch of the basilar artery. It winds around the cerebral peduncle forming a curve whose shape is rather variable. The two posterior cerebral arteries fix the boundaries of the brain stem in an oblique direction upwards and backwards. In this fashion they course into the ambiens cistern on the internal concavity of the temporal lobe parallel to the basal vein. Consequently they are in direct contact with the hippocampus and the internal gyri of the temporal lobe. One can make out segment P_1, or precommunicating one, a short trunk which measures 0,5 to 1 cm in length. The posterior thalamo-perforating arteries arise in this segment. Segment P_2, or post-communicating one, corresponds to the upper and lateral peduncular portion as far as the region above the quadrigeminal body where the left and right arteries converge. Segments P_3 and P_4 concern the temporo-occipital area, lying outside the mesencephalon, object of our study. Very often segment P_2 describes a small concave curve towards the exterior at the level of the lateral mesencephalic sulcus. The minimal distance between the two arteries at the end of segment P_2 corresponds on the one hand to the quadrigeminal cistern and on the other hand to the free edge of the tentorium. In principle, the frontal distance between the posterior cerebral arteries gives the width of the brain stem. However, this notion is not always valid since it is of no great importance in diagnosing a peduncular atrophy. Such an atrophy easily occurs without shifting of the posterior cerebral artery. We frequently view quite normal arteriograms in severe cases of peduncular atrophy (Fig. 7).

We measured the maximum and minimum distance between the posterior cerebral arteries and noted these measurements in the table of Fig. 8.

The minimum distance measured at the level of the free margin of the tentorium varies from 1 to 3 cms, while the maximum distance measures 3,5 to 5,5 cms. These variations are too great to furnish us an indication for a diagnosis. We have utilized a technique of photographic summation to establish these variations. Thus was produced Fig. 9 which shows the variations in the course of the posterior cerebral arteries in normal cases. The normal frontal view is characterized by the symmetry and the morphology of the artery. However, this symmetry is not a perfect one in that the artery departs from the midline in an identical fashion on both sides but often at a different level. The shape of the curve is of great importance since segmentary straightness is a major element in the diagnosis of peduncular tumours (Figs. 95–105).

Lateral View. The two posterior cerebral arteries are superimposed. In fact, the prepeduncular segment (segment P_1) is seen tangentially, thus its image adds no new information to what is already known. The second segment, which is lateropeduncular (P_2) and quite visible, is concave upwards. This segment, however, is oriented towards the axis of the posterior cerebral artery, that is, towards the line which connects the tuberculum sellae to a point midway between the lambdoidal suture and the internal occipital protuberance. We have encountered great variations in the angle formed by the basilar trunk and segment P_2 in 90 normal cases. Fig. 10 represents the superimposition of the tracings of these 90 cases and shows the wide dispersion of the angle.

2. The Posterior Thalamo-Perforating Arteries
(Figs. 11–14)

These arteries are of a relatively thin calibre, generally badly distinguishable in a frontal view, and more easily indentifiable in a lateral view. Among our cases we have encountered approximately 5 normal radioanatomical types. These variants are illustrated in Fig. 13. In the majority of cases (48%) three arteries seem to arise from the upper extremity of the basilar artery, prolonging its axis while taking an upward and backward direction. A slightly sharper inclination with respect to the basilar artery is rarer (8%). More often one or two arteries emerging from the posterior cerebral artery have been observed (36%). These arteries are always more or less tortuous and their angiographic identification is easy. We shall see that straightnesses or shiftings can be easily viewed in pathological cases. Cases where posterior thalamo-perforating arteries take the shape of a single channel, 0,5 to 1 cm in length, and having terminal ramifications, are smaller in number.

18

Viewed frontally, these arteries are sometimes identifiable in normal cases due to their para-medial topography. In pathological cases the opacification may be greater, due to intra-cranial hypertension or to arteriosclerosis.

3. The Colliculi Quadrigemini and Corpori Geniculati Arteries (Figs. 15–17)

These arteries have been dissected. They are often of high calibre, so much so that one would expect an angiographic view as good as the one of the posterior thalamo-perforating arteries. Actually this is not so, since these arteries are rarely opacified in routine angiographies. Furthermore, their identification is easy only if the posterior thalamo-perforating arteries and the choroidal arteries are both opacified. We have encountered two morphological types, one where a common channel divides in two branches, another where two branches stem immediately on either side (20%). We have never had good views of these arteries in frontal or axial projections of normal cases.

4. Posterior Choroidal Arteries

In the mesencephalon, these are the most important collateral branches of the posterior cerebral artery. We have referred to an important bibliography concerning them. Dissections performed in collaboration with Dr. Held in Strasbourg have shown us a great variety in the lay-out of these arteries. In spite of often contradictory discussions on the part of anatomists, we must establish a classification suited to the needs of angiographic diagnosis. For practical reasons, the two classical groups, the posterior medial choroidal and the lateral posterior choroidal, must be separated. Any other approach risks to be too theoretical and devoid of usefulness in angiography.

a) The Medial Posterior Choroidal Arteries (Figs. 18–25)

Frontal View. Under normal conditions, this artery is rarely visible, in which case it appears as a relatively thin vessel, separated from the prepeduncular segment of the posterior cerebral artery and winding with it around the brain stem to attain finally the pineal region near the midline. When this artery is well opacified in a frontal view, pathological conditions such as feeding of a malformation, or a tumour, or intra-cranial hypertension are certainly to be suspected.

Lateral View. A vertebral angiogram permits the viewing of the two medial posterior choroidal arteries. The left and right artery describe double anterior concave curves as in a figure 3 The lower curve corresponds to the lateral peduncular course. Before attaining the pineal region, the artery reaches a point in an anterior direction in the lateral mesencephalic sulcus. This point marks the beginning of the upper anterior concave curve. The posterior segment of this curve corresponds to the lateral pineal region. This segment ends in an anterior direction. Its length depends on angiographic conditions, such as the size of the artery, and technical conditions. Generally the artery divides itself into two branches which are distinguishable in certain angiograms (Fig. 18). A main trunk runs forward into the choroidal plexus of the IIIrd ventricle to complete the upper concavity of the figure 3. A secondary branch, less visible in angiograms, takes a variable course to reach the choroidal plexus of the lateral ventricle. In our illustrations, the medial choroidal arteries have a quite fixed topography in the anterior portion of Löfgren's diagram. From a morphological point of view, one does not always encounter a figure 3. Fig. 22 sums up the types of shapes that we have observed, notably:

—an "undulated" shape which does not really take the form of a figure 3 in 40% of cases. It is possible to confuse this type of artery with the lateral posterior choroidal artery. The application of Löfgren's diagram, and measurement of the distance given in Figs. 31, 32 and 33 permit to establish the exact topography of the artery.

—a typical figure 3 which leaves no doubt as to the identification of the artery: 40% of cases.

—a special kind of Fig. 3 whose upper concavity is wide and whose lower concavity is short and deep in 20% of cases.

When the pineal gland is well calcified, its relations to the artery can be easily established. These relations, as illustrated in Fig. 44, are important, since they permit to formulate clearly a criterion of normality in arterial-pineal relations. Very often angiography is poor in the mesencephalon. If the normal medial posterior choroidal artery is viewable, this constitutes proof that a mass lesion is absent. Other arteries, and in particular the lateral posterior choroidal arteries, are less often opacified.

b) The Lateral Posterior Choroidal Arteries (Figs. 26–30)

Frontal View. These arteries are rarely visible in a frontal view. In cases where they are identifiable, they can be seen to emerge from the lateral peduncular portion of the posterior cerebral artery. For a short distance they accompany the posterior cerebral artery, leaving it progressively to take a lateral course. We have never been able to identify more than one lateral posterior choroidal artery in an angiogram, although dissection reveals up to four of these on each side. When this artery is greatly visible in a frontal view, there is suspicion of pathological hypertrophy: feeding of a malformation, tumour, or intracranial hypertension.

Lateral View. The number of lateral choroidal arteries is extremely variable. Depending on the case, 2 to 6 overlapping arteries are visible in a lateral view. These arteries describe a large anterior concave curve when they wind around the brain stem. They run into the ambient cisterns and cross the choroidal fissure. A lateral branch attains the choroidal plexus of the temporal lobe and of the lateral ventricle. Another branch goes around the pulvinar describing a large anterior concave curve which terminates in the trigone where it forms an anastomotic network with the anterior choroidal artery. Its anterior concave course follows the posterior and superior margin of Löfgren's diagram (Figs. 31, 32, 33).

5. Posterior Pericallosal Artery (Figs. 34 and 38)

We could identify this artery only in a lateral projection. It issues from the posterior cerebral artery not far from the midline. In about 50% of cases, it takes a forward direction for a short distance and then curves around the splenium in an anteriorly directed concave curve. In the remaining 50% of cases, it immediately describes a large concavity around the splenium. In Figs. 34 and 37 we show rare pictures of transversal sinuosities of this artery.

The main topographic characteristic of this artery is its position outside and behind Löfgren's diagram. Löfgren's diagram (Fig. 33) is particularly useful in distinguishing the pericallosal artery from the posterior lateral choroidal artery. Since both arteries often have a similar morphology, only their topographic characteristics permit their differentiation. This is easy under normal conditions but becomes very difficult in certain pathological cases, especially when the posterior lateral choroidal artery is shifted backwards (Fig. 36).

6. Pericallosal Arterial Circle (Figs. 34–38)

Under normal conditions, the anastomosis of anterior and posterior pericallosal arteries forms an arterial circle which is seldom seen. Under pathological conditions, on the contrary, this circle becomes functional and can be filled with contrast medium, as shown in Fig. 35. This pericallosal circle can act as collateral circulation, especially in cases of thrombosis of the anterior cerebral artery.

We shall point out later on that a backward shifting of the posterior lateral choroidal artery can bring about a superimposition of its distal segment with the extremity of the anterior pericallosal artery. Consequently this gives a false picture of the pericallosal circle (Fig. 36).

Dissection reveals that this artery varies in its course and in its collaterals. Fig. 38 shows a case with two posterior pericallosal arteries having different dispositions on the left and on the right.

7. Capillarography in the Final Phase of the Arteriogram (Fig. 40)

Capillarography has contributed to the progress achieved in angiography due to the method of subtraction which permits a contrast medium to be seen during the capillary phase. In practice, the execution of an image through subtraction is relatively easy when technical conditions are good: seriographic timing, immobilization of the patient, amount of contrast medium injected and photographic technique. We have utilized solely a lateral projection in the capillarographic study of the final phase of the arteriogram. It has been observed that the region of the pulvinar is quite rapidly opacified, almost at the end of the arterial phase. The opacification of the posterior thalamus is just as dense during the arterial phase as it is during the venous phase. It appears that this thalamic opacification is all the more intense when venous drainage is slow. We shall see further on that capillarography of the vertebro-basilar system is all the denser when there exists increased intra-cranial pressure, that is, an obstacle in venous drainage. Although these observations remain theoretical, they have fashioned our practical attitude in the execution of views using subtraction in the capillarography of the mesencephalon.

It is necessary to take several views during the capillary phase and to compress the jugular veins and the V_1 segment of the other vertebral artery during the injection to retard venous reflux.

Capillarography in the final phase of the arteriogram presents some difficulties as our experience is still limited. We shall list here a few conclusions we have reached during our angiographic experiences:

1. The anterior margin of the opacified thalamic parenchyma is well outlined by the posterior thalamo-perforating arteries.

2. The thalamic parenchyma is opacified sooner than the choroidal plexus of the IIIrd ventricle, that is, to say, there is a clear difference in circulatory speed between these two areas.

3. The posterior limit of the thalamus is not clearly outlined but corresponds approximately to the course of the postero-lateral choroidal artery.

8. The Relations between the Pineal Gland and the Choroidal Arteries (Fig. 44)

Viewed anatomically, the postero-medial choroidal artery courses parallel to the posterior cerebral artery, turns when it reaches the brain stem and crosses the quadrigeminal cistern to terminate in the plexus of the IIIrd ventricle. This artery is located slightly outside and lateral to the pineal gland which it supplies with small branches. In a lateral angiographic view, the topographic relations of the pineal gland and the postero-medial and lateral choroidal arteries are variable. It has generally been observed that the postero-medial choroidal artery courses in a double anterior concave curve remindful of a figure 3. The inferior concavity of this artery projects itself on the middle and posterior region of the pineal gland, after which it courses forward. At this point the anterior pole of the pineal gland coincides with the anterior point formed by the junction of the two half circles in the figure 3.

However, depending on the different morphological variants of the postero-medial choroidal artery, this topographic disposition can vary. Thus the pineal gland can be found slightly in front of or behind this artery. It is sometimes slightly visible in the inferior concavity of the artery. Generally it is visible a few millimeters above the middle portion of the posterior cerebral artery.

The close relationship of the postero-medial choroidal artery and the pineal gland is constant. The distance between its external margin and the gland varies between 4 and 5 mm.

In half axial projections the pineal gland is located on the midline. When the postero-medial choroidal artery is visible, something which rarely happens, it is located 4–6 mm to the side of the pineal gland.

Normal Radioanatomy of the Veins

Normal venous radioanatomy of the veins of the mesencephalic region and their principal normal variations are illustrated in Figs. 45–75. The characteristics of each of these veins are outlined in this chapter in order to facilitate the interpretation of pathological cases in the mesencephalic region and its immediate surrounding area.

The Basal Vein

This vein is the principal angiographic venous element in the mesencephalon. The two basal veins outline the upper lateral part of the mesencephalon and because of this fact have the same diagnostic value as the ambient cisterns in pneumo-encephalography.

Origin. Three venous currents in confluence are at the origin of the basal vein:

—Henle's anterior vein, which is formed by the anterior pericallosal vein, the orbital vein and the olfactive vein;

—the deep middle cerebral vein or insular vein;

—the lower strial vein formed by several nuclear and capsular veins.

An anterior communicating vein joins the two basal veins at their origin and matches functionally the anterior communicating artery.

Tributaries. The nomenclature of the numerous tributary veins permits an inventory of the regions drained. These are:

—the interpeduncular veins, formed by the chiasmal, tuberian and mammillar veins;

—the pontomesencephalic veins;

—the plexuses of the lateral ventricle, known as ventricular veins;

—the strial veins;

—hippocampal veins;

—geniculate veins;

—peduncular veins;

—lateral mesencephalic veins;

—thalamic veins.

Only a few of these veins are sufficiently well defined to be of practical value in angiography.

Course. The vein courses from the optochiasmic and crural cisterns through the interpeduncular and lateral cisterns to the cistern of the great vein of Galen.

Finishing Point. The great vein of Galen.

Regions Drained. The aforementioned tributaries designate the regions drained. In carotid angiography the two basal veins drain the contrast fluid under the following conditions: when the anterior cerebral artery supplies the opposite hemisphere; or when the two anterior cerebral arteries are opacified by a common trunk or a functional anterior communicating artery; or when Hendon's interbasal anastomosis is functional. In vertebral angiography the two basal veins are opacified in the same manner when the two posterior cerebral arteries receive an equal amount of contrast medium.

a) Normal Roentgenographic Anatomy of the Basal Vein during Selective Carotid Angiography

The basal vein is a large venous channel visible in frontal and lateral projections. Its calibre is equal to or higher than the internal cerebral vein. In fronto-suboccipital projections, its origin is found at the level of the internal auditory meatus and one can often distinguish interbasilar anastomosis. In a lateral projection its origin is found over and in front of the sella turcica. Its course may be divided into two segments going in different directions:

—*the anterior segment :* approximatively parallel to Reid's basal line, it goes from the origin to point L, which we establish at the junction of the interpeduncular pontomesencephalic veins and the anterior horizontal and posterior oblique parts of the basal vein. Since in carotid angiography the interpeduncular and ponto-mesencephalic veins are not opacified, point L matches the point of the angle formed by the two segments of the basal vein. In a frontal view point L matches the most external point of the basal vein at the brainstem level.

—*the posterior segment :* extends from point L (the anterior-inferior lateral peduncular region) to the great vein of Galen running through the ambient cistern next to the posterior cerebral artery. Often point L shows a change in the calibre of the vein since the posterior segment is larger than the anterior.

b) Normal Roentgenographic Anatomy of the Basal Vein in Selective Vertebral Angiography

Lateral View. In this view the posterior segment only is visible. The tributaries from point L, that is the interpeduncular and pontomesencephalic veins, are also distinguishable. The principal tributary from point L, that is, the anterior segment of the basal vein, is missing, as it depends entirely on the carotidial system.

Frontal View. In this view one rarely distinguishes the basal vein in its entirety. When it is well opacified it is easily identified from the midline (the interpeduncular vein) to the great vein of Galen which it joins while circumscribing the cerebral peduncle (Fig. 48). When the basal vein is opacified on both sides, and that interbasal anastomosis is functional, one can distinguish a continuous course outlining the limits of the cerebral trunk in the peduncular region. At times the basal vein is missing in a carotid angiogram while it is opacified in a vertebral angiogram. In these cases it is very difficult to determine whether it is the posterior segment of the basal vein which does not communicate with the anterior segment or whether it is the posterior mesencephalic vein.

c) Normal Roentgenographic Anatomy of the Basal Vein in Brachial Angiography on the Same Side

Retrograde angiography through the right brachial artery opacifies simultaneously both the carotid and the vertebral arteries. In these cases the entire basal vein and frequently both veins are opacified.

In a frontal view the basal vein comes out better from the left side since it is partially hidden on the right by the overlying of the other veins of the posterior fossa. In vertebro-carotidian angiography, the opacification of the two basal veins is increased on the one hand by anterior chiasmic anastomosis and on the other hand by posterior peduncular anastomosis.

Roentgenographic Anatomic Variants of the Basal Vein

Absence of the Basal Vein (Fig. 50). This is frequent in carotid angiography. The contrast medium in the basal region is drained by the other veins. The possibilities of this form of drainage are numerous.

Absence of the Anterior Segment of the Basal Vein (Fig. 50b). The entire portion situated in front of point L is missing. The region is drained towards the sphenoparietal sinus of Brechet and towards the cavernous sinus. The posterior segment of the basal vein is present and communicates with the superior petrosal sinus via the mesencephalic vein. In this case, the posterior segment of the basal vein is called the posterior mesencephalic vein. Its blood is fed only through the vertebral artery.

Absence of the Posterior Segment of the Basal Vein (Figs. 53A and B). This is an anomaly which Huang described under the term "anastomotic lateral mesencephalic vein".

Outflow Anomalies (Figs. 51 and 52). Instead of flowing into the great vein of Galen, the basal vein flows into the lateral sinus or into the straight sinus. Hedon points out the possibility of outflow of the basal vein into a cerebellar vein.

The Interpeduncular Veins

These veins form a venous plexus in the interpeduncular space. They connect the left basal vein with the right one and usually join the pontomesencephalic vein to flow with it into the homo-lateral basal vein at point L. In certain cases, the interpeduncular veins flow into the homo-lateral branch of the pontomesence-phalic vein which does not drain into the basal vein but rather into the venous plexus of the clivus. The interpeduncular venous plexus is formed by internal and inferior peduncular veins such as the tuberian veins, the mammillary veins, the thalamic and hypothalamic veins (Fig. 57).

The Pontomesencephalic Vein

This vein drains blood from the pons of Varole and runs on its anterior aspect near the midline. It drains towards the superior petrosal sinus, the plexus of the clivus and the basal vein (Figs. 58 and 59). Because of this, this vein has an anastomotic role among the different regions. The regular calibre of this vein seen in a lateral angiographic view confirms its anastomotic character. The topography and shape of the ponto-mesencephalic vein is characteristic, outlining the posterior wall of the pontine cistern which forms an anteriorly convex curve behind the dorsum sellae. This curve has an italic "S" shape whose upper concavity is formed by the interpeduncular veins while the inferior convexity contains the ponto-mesencephalic veins. The highest and most anterior point matches the perforating anterior space. The upper part of the "S" corresponds to the first and second segment described by Huang (1968). The inferior convexity belongs entirely to the pontomesencephalic vein proper. In its prepontine course, the pontomesencephalic vein is medial and single. It divides to form a "Y" shape communicating with the right and left petrosal veins (transversal prepontine veins). Sometimes the two dividing branches appear in lateral phlebograms as small veins running into the petrosal opacity. The pontomesencephalic vein communicates with the prebulbar vein and the premedular venous system.

The Lateral Mesencephalic Vein

This particular vein is of interest because of its location in a zone of transition between the subtentorial and supratentorial areas. Unfortunately the vein is not always visible. Howewer a perfectly acceptable image is obtained in 30% of cases (Figs. 60–62).

Origin : superior petrosal sinus.

Course : the lateral mesencephalic sulcus. Thus the vein is an excellent guidemark to delimit the basis pedunculis and tegmentum.

Tributaries : its tributaries are usually invisible in angiography. Their calibre is small and they issue from the brachium conjonctivum.

Finishing Point : it terminates in the basal vein at an angle of 80° which opens forward and downward.

Angiographically, the lateral mesencephalic vein is generally not well opacified by carotid injection but we observed cases of good opacification (Fig. 62).

Vertebral Angiography :

frontal—we have never been able to identify indisputably the lateral mesencephalic vein in frontal projections in normal cases.

lateral—the vein flows into the basal vein approximately midway between the junction of the pontomesencephalic vein and the precentral vein. Its course is more or less straight towards the petrosal sinus. It forms an imperfect right angle, opening forward and downward. Its junction with the basal vein is clearly located behind point L. The calibre of the lateral mesencephalic vein is usually small, however expansions can be observed which are limited to the mesencephalic vein. In these cases it probably has an anastomotic role between the normal basal vein and the petrosal sinus (Fig. 61).

The Anterior Great Cerebellar Vein

This vein is an embryonic vestige which, due to its anastomotic function, permits the joining of the superior petrosal sinus with the great vein of Galen. It is divided into three segments (Figs. 54, 55A and B).

—an inferior segment corresponding to the petrosal vein,

—a middle segment corresponding to the lateral mesencephalic vein,

—a posterior segment corresponding to the posterior part of the embryonic anterior cerebellar vein.

We have observed this topography in three cases.

Lateral Anastomic Mesencephalic Vein (Figs. 53 A and B)

Huang has provided the angiographic image of this variant. The anomaly described by Padget presents an absence of the posterior segment of the basal vein, in which case a large lateral mesencephalic vein communicates in front with the anterior part of the basal vein, and in back with the superior petrosal sinus.

The Mesencepalic-Petrosal-Hemispheric System

We reproduce here the image of a venous anastomosis between Galen's system and the lateral sinus. This vein is formed successively by the posterior part of the basal vein—the lateral mesencephalic vein—the petrosal vein and a hemispheric cerebellar vein (Fig. 70).

The Precentral Cerebellar Vein

Huang and Wolff made a precise and original study of the precentral cerebellar vein in 1966. The authors insisted on the fact that little information could be gathered from the description of these veins in classical anatomical works.

The precentral cerebellar vein originates in the fissure which separates the lingula from the central lobule. Medial sagittal pneumostratigraphy does not show this fissure in all its depth. Since gas cannot penetrate to the depth of the fissure, only the entrance is generally seen. The precentral cerebellar vein is formed by the union of two symmetrical tributaries emerging from each side in the lateral extension of the precentral cerebellar fissure. They run medially within this fissure to join one another in the midline. This lateral extension is limited by the anterior and middle cerebellar peduncle and is called the interpeduncular cerebellar space. The precentral cerebellar vein courses in the depths of the precentral fissure; in the first portion it runs forward and upward to reach the surface of the cerebellum, just in front of the anterior aspect of the IVth ventricle. When the vein leaves the precentral fissure it turns backward and upward at some distance from the vermis and joins the posterior end of the great vein of Galen at its junction with the straight sinus. The venous topography we have described should be considered as a prototype subject to variations. Often the two tributaries do not unite in the precentral cerebellar fissure but continue as individual trunks in an upward direction for a variable distance before joining. Thus each courses separately to the great vein of Galen or to the internal cerebral vein. These two tributaries often communicate with each other by transverse connections called communicating veins. The length of the medial venous trunk varies depending on the level of junction of its tributaries.

In a *frontal view* the precentral vein is often difficult to recognize because of the overlying of the internal cerebral veins, of the great vein of Galen and of the medial vermian vein. Sometimes the venous tributaries and the single central trunk appear as an inverted "y". This corresponds to the sides of the IVth ventricle. A frontal projection of this ventricle in pneumography is of great assistance to the neuroradiologist in identifying these veins. The single trunk or the paired precentral veins course on the midline or the paramedial line to reach finally the great vein of Galen (Fig. 63).

In a *lateral projection* using subtraction the precentral cerebellar vein appears clearly in the shape of an italic "s". The lower horizontal portion courses in the central-lingular fissure. The intermediate portion runs in front of the central lobule. The upper portion, slightly concave anteriorly, generally reaches the posterior part of the great vein of Galen near its junction with the right sinus. Though the italic "S" is the usual shape taken by the vein, there sometimes exist other variations which depend on the form of the cerebellar vermis. Huang describes a variation whose shape consists of a single trunk formed by the junction of the upper vermian vein with the precentral vein. The normal topography of the precentral vein in a frontal projection lies on the midline. It should be emphasized that, according to Huang, the lateral view of the vein corresponds to the "C–C" point in the central-collicular region, that is, at the union of the IVth ventricle with the aqueduct of Sylvius. If needed, this point can be used as a guiding mark in the same fashion as those established by Lysholm and Twinning. The precentral vein is a single and medial vessel, consequently it points out midline shiftings in spite of the overlying of the great cerebral vein and the straight sinus in a frontal projection.

A lateral projection is more useful, since the vein marks the limit between the mesencephalon above and the cerebellum below (Fig. 75). It indicates the direction of growth of expansive lesions (Figs. 106–119). Laterally it forms an angle which we shall call collicular since its lateral projection embraces the quadrigeminal tubercules.

The Paracentral Vein or the Lateral Precentral Vein

Huang and Wolf give a good example of this vein in a frontal projection. It courses upwards to join the great vein of Galen. This paired vessel runs along its entire length on the paramidline. In a frontal projection there can be no confusion with the precentral vein; however, in a lateral projection its topography is similar to the precentral vein though it is shorter and straighter.

The Superior Vermian Vein or Huang's Supraculminate Vein

Origin : It is formed by the junction of several branches whose topography and calibre vary. These emerge from the cerebellar hemisphere.

Course : It flows into the superior vermian system above the culmen.

Finishing Point : It terminates in the great vein of Galen slightly forward of the precentral vein.

Variants (Fig. 64) *:*—Junction with the precental vein forming a common trunk which then flows into the great vein of Galen.
—Junction with the basal vein.
—a large perivermian vein formed above by the superior vermian vein and below by the inferior vermian vein.

The superior vermian vein is of slight interest in mesencephalic angiography. However, it delimits the posterior boundary in the area of expansion of mesencephalic tumours.

The Marginal Cerebellar Vein

This vein was studied by Rosa and Viale in 1968. It is plainly visible in a lateral projection, and its identification is facilitated by its undulated course following an oblique upward and backward direction. It connects the mesencephalic lateral vein with the superior vermian vein, and often overlies the course of the precentral vein.

Veins in the Dural and Tentorial Walls of the Posterior Fossa

These are numerous and variable. In angiographic examination one can distinguish:

1.—a vein above the lateral sinus which courses parallel to the sinus.

2.—lateral veins which flow into the lateral or sigmoid sinus.
3.—a vein on the free edge of the cerebellum's tent.
4.—the basal plexus which extends from the cavernous sinus to the superior petrosal sinus.
5.—the occipital plexus which extends from the basal plexus to the internal vertebral plexus and the torcular around the occipital foramen.

Only the vein on the free edge of the cerebellum's tent and the upper portion of the basal plexus is of interest in mesencephalic angiography (Fig. 65).

Ventricular Veins

We observed a normal (Fig. 69) and a pathological case (Fig.111) of strongly opacified ventricular veins.

Capillarography in the Venous Phase

The capillarographic view in the venous phase (Fig. 71) differs greatly from that in the arterial phase (Fig. 40). Contrast in the venous phase is generally more marked and thalamic vessels can be better observed. These usually consist of large veins which join either the internal cerebral vein or the basal vein. The stasis in the posterior fossa easily produces such a sharp capillarography because venous drainage is difficult and slow. This stasis is particularly observed in cases of tumours of the mesencephalic region (Figs. 93, 127 and 128).

The Relationship of the Pineal Gland and the Veins

A study of the relationship between the pineal gland and the veins can be made only in lateral projections. In frontal projections, the degree of angulation of the central ray and the degree of flexion of the patient's head influence much too greatly the position of the vascular elements with respect to the pineal body.

The calcified pineal gland is usually located in the angle formed by the posterior segment of the internal cerebral vein above the distal segment of Rosenthal's basal vein below (Fig. 73).

The appraisal of the pineal body and its relations depends primarily on its degree of calcification. As a matter of fact, we can appraise solely the calcifications, which usually represent a part, more or less extended, of the gland.

A second factor for appraisal is the centering of the lateral angiographic image. Inaccuracy can cause slight variations in the lateral projection of these elements in the radiogram. The distance between the internal cerebral vein and the pineal gland varies under normal conditions between 3 and 5 mm, whereas the distance between the calcified pineal gland and Rosenthal's basal vein varies between 5 and 8 mm. At times a third venous landmark appears under the form of the posterior cerebral vein (or the superior thalamic vein) which follows a parallel course 4 mm below the internal cerebral vein.

The posterior segment of this vein is in direct contact with the calcifications of the pineal gland, which are immediately localised below. These vascular relations vary depending on the localisation of the intracranial mass.

1. Tumours of the pineal region increase the distance between the veins and the calcifications, as the tumoral expansions displace the internal cerebral vein upwards and the basal vein downwards.

2. Hemispherical tumours as well as hematomas influence these relationships in a different manner:

a) Convexity hematomas as well as mass expansions depress the course of the internal cerebral vein and thus draws them closer to the pineal gland decreasing the distance between them.

b) Infratemporal tumours lift the basal vein thus diminishing its distance.

Venous Topogram

The relationship among the various deep veins is outlined in Fig. 75. Topographic considerations are of great practical value in diagnosing tumoral expansions. The facts reported in this figure are sufficiently explicit of themselves to go without commentary.

Pathological Findings

Tumours of the Pineal Region

Our experience with tumours will be outlined here in the order usually followed by neurosurgeons. In actual fact we could proceed strictly from the neuroradiological point of view by describing the localisation and the angiographic signs which acquaint us with the nature of the tumour. This would not substantially change the traditional manner which permits us to distinguish tumours of the pineal region. A mass expansion in this region can be localised whereas its precise origin remains enigmatic. Vertebral angiography carried out in 10 cases permits us the following observations:

1. Arterial Displacements in the Lateral Projection

As in Fig. 78, it is quite clear that the posterior medial choroidal artery is displaced backwards. The application of Löfgren's diagram verifies this displacement. In cases where the posterior chorioidal arteries as a group are largely displaced, as in Fig. 76, it is difficult to distinguish the posterior medial choroidal artery. The additional fact that this artery loses its characteristic figure "3" shape increases the difficulty, though the curves are sometimes faintly outlined.

—The most anteriorly situated artery is the medial posterior choroidal artery, although exceptions may be encountered. Usually the medial and lateral arteries group themselves in a network which falls behind Löfgren's diagram.

—The medial artery arises from the posterior cerebral artery more forwards than the lateral artery. When both points of emergence are clearly visible, the identification of the medial artery is easy.

When a pineal tumour extends largely to one side, it displaces mainly the lateral posterior artery (Fig. 77), which may be located behind the posterior pericallosal artery. In such cases it is difficult to distinguish a pineal tumour from one belonging to the posterior thalamic region.

In all cases of pineal tumours, the posterior choroidal arteries fall outside Löfgren's diagram. This displacement may be slight posteriorly, but it is always important in a postero-superior direction.

The posterior thalamo-perforating arteries may be pushed forward, straightened, or present a posterior concavity. When these arteries appear in the angiogram, they are enlarged either due to intra-cranial hypertension or to the presence of a tumour. The posterior thalamo-perforating arteries indicate a tumoral extension to the thalamus.

The arteries of the colliculi quadrigemini and corpori geniculati may participate in the blood supply of a tumour. They are then hypertrophied and in consequence quite visible, whereas they are only slightly opacified in normal cases (Fig. 78).

The different figures illustrate the importance of backward displacement of the posterior choroidal arteries compared to the normal range. This backward displacement, measured on our angiograms, is relatively slight compared to the normal. Accordingly, these angiographic deformations are less pronounced as pneumographic alterations, so much so that we feel that the pinealoma develops particularly forward in the IIIrd ventricle.

2. Arterial Displacements in the Frontal Projection

Two types of arterial displacements are to be noted:

a) Rigidity of the posterior cerebral arteries in the pineal region. This segmentary rigidity is at times sufficiently pronounced to be of value in diagnosis. Such a deformation is the result of a relatively important tumour. In cases where a pineal tumour is voluminous, the posterior cerebral arteries can also be displaced laterally. Average-sized pineal tumours do not, however, cause such displacements and would not fall out of the norm reproduced in Fig. 8.

b) The hammock sign we described in 1968 in Cologne. This sign is rarer (2 out of 10 cases) and is not characteristic of a pinealoma but recurs also in retromesencephalic masses such as medial meningiomas of the free edge of the tentorium. It consists of an abnormal elongated artery which extends transversally across the midline in an upward concave curvature, outlining the lower margin of the tumour. In our two cases it was difficult to define the origin of this abnormal artery. It can issue from a posterior cerebral, posterior choroidal or superior cerebellar artery of anastomised transversal pineal branches of the postero-medial choroidal arteries. Fig. 82 illustrates the hammock sign.

3. Spontaneously Opacified Tumoral Vascularisation

Spontaneous opacification was observed in only two of the 10 cases in our hands (Figs. 79 and 81). It concerned malignant tumours in both cases. As in other cerebral tumours, the correlation between tumoral vessels and malignancy is variable. In one case a tumoral stain provoked a late opacification of the entire tumoral mass.

4. Avascular Image of the Tumour

In 8 of our cases no tumoral vessels appear. In only one of our cases was there a peritumoral stain sufficiently marked to reveal the avascular nature of a pineal tumour through the use of contrast (Fig. 83). We are aware of the radiographic pitfalls of subtraction, but we feel nonetheless that in the area of avascular tumours there is a further possibility for angiographic diagnosis.

5. Calcification of the Pineal Gland

Calcifications of the pineal body have been of no help in any of our observations. None of our proven tumours were calcified. In one case, not proven anatomically, the calcifications were rather numerous in the pineal area, displacing backwards the posterior choroidal arteries. It was probably the case of a small asymptomatic pinealoma (Fig. 84).

6. Arterial Hypertrophy

In all our cases the posterior choroidal arteries are enlarged. This arterial hypertrophy explains the good visibility of such small vessels as the colliculi quadrigemini and corpori geniculati arteries, otherwise invisible in normal subjects.

7. Venous Displacement

Venous displacement is as marked as arterial displacement and is concomitant to an alteration of the walls and the diameter of the vein. This permits to define the tumoral nature of the expansion through angiography.

The venous topogram in Fig. 75 permits us to localise the pineal body in the angle formed by the internal cerebral vein and the basal vein. It is at this level that one normally encounters the calcified pineal gland (Fig. 73).

Pineal expansion takes its departure in this area and causes the following phenomena, as seen in Figs. 76, 79, 81, 85.:

—an elevation of the terminal portion of the internal cerebral vein near its junction with the great vein of Galen. This part of the vein becomes rigid and its concave course becomes exaggerated.

—variable modifications of the basal vein on one side or on both sides. Thus the course of the basal vein becomes rigid, is sometimes displaced backwards, or its visibility is cut off. The more the basal vein is subject to alterations, the greater is the tumour or its infiltrations. Fig. 76 clearly shows a venous hammock bordering the postero-inferior margin of the tumour. This however is an exception. More often the vein is dislocated or cut off at the level of point "L".

It is in this region that anomalies are markedly visible in a lateral projection (Figs. 79 and 81). As illustrated in these figures, the entire dilatation of the posterior thalamic veins is visible only in a lateral projection. This important indication does not necessarily imply an encroachment of the thalamus. Blood from the pineal tumour can drain normally in the terminal portion, without its having infiltrated the posterior portion of the thalamus.

Our angiographic experience is based on the observation of 10 pineal tumours, from which three particular types can be pointed out:

1. *The case of a very large malignant tumour* accompanied by arterial and venous alterations and sometimes late impregnation of the tumoral mass. Angiography in itself suffices to arrive at a diagnosis.

2. *The case of a middle-sized tumour* 2 cms in diameter. The venous and arterial modifications are marked but the best indications are had by the double contrast: angiographic and encephalic. It has been observed that a forward displacement in the wall of the IIIrd ventricle is more marked than the backward displacement of the arteries and veins.

3. *The case of a small tumour* less than 1 cm in diameter is likely to go unobserved on an angiogram when it does not entail a spontaneous opacification. It can be placed in evidence negatively, that is, in an avascular zone through subtraction.

Tumours of the Posterior Thalamus

The mesencephalic region is often infiltrated by expansions of posterior thalamic tumoral masses. The network of arteries and veins in this area forecasts the early modifications provoked by tumoral masses. In actual practice it is often difficult to recognize a posterior thalamic localisation since the tumour has often infiltrated the thalamus or the peduncles when the patients come for angiographic examination. Sometimes, however, we do find a mass occupying essentially the posterior thalamus, which is entirely supplied by the vertebro-basilar system. Vertebral angiography must be performed to arrive at a diagnosis.

1. Arteries

The interpretation of a frontal angiogram provides little information on thalamic tumours since displacements are usually antero-posterior. Lateral expansions of posterior thalamic tumours are not revealed in frontal views. It is for these reasons that we shall limit our observations of pure thalamic tumours to lateral angiograms.

a) Postero-Lateral Choroidal Artery

This artery in its relations with the posterior thalamus provides the keystone in angiographic diagnosis of posterior thalamic tumours. The increase in the radius of its curvature is a major sign when the tumour is limited to the posterior thalamus. A lateral projection in its initial phase shows solely a backward displacement of the postero-lateral choroidal artery. This displacement is the opposite of that produced by a pinealoma, which is initially limited to the postero-medial choroidal artery.

Fig. 104 illustrates these observations in the case of a unilateral posterior thalamic tumour. When a tumour has embodied the artery, it is deformed and sometimes displaced frontwards, as is the case in Fig. 87. Under these conditions the artery is no longer a landmark in the measurement of tumoral expansions.

b) The Postero-Medial Choroidal Artery

The characteristic figure "3" shape persists at the beginning of the tumoral evolution. It is only later that this artery follows the displacement of the postero-lateral choroidal artery.

c) The Colliculi Quadrigemini and Corporis Callosi Arteries

When the tumour grows to a certain size, these arteries take part in the tumoral blood supply. They become hypertrophied, thus visible. Sometimes they are rigid and displaced towards the front (Figs. 88 and 93).

d) The Posterior Thalamic Perforating Arteries

In a late stage these hypertrophied arteries either become rigid when they are embodied in the tumour, or are displaced towards the front under tumoral pressure. They are then visible in a frontal view where their hypertrophy alone leads to suspect a tumour of the thalamus (Figs. 88, 93).

2. Capillarography

In spite of the good indications obtained in observing the arteries and particularly the veins, capillarography of a pathological thalamus is of interest. The normal capillarographic view of the thalamus is had in Figs. 40 and 71. In cases of tumour, vascular opacity takes an abnormal form and increases in volume. Capillarography is an important contribution since it complements classical angiography.

Capillarography alone permits a direct viewing of the tumour. All the morphological tumoral degrees can be observed: from an intrathalamic tumoral zone (Fig. 92A), to the large butterfly-shaped opacity of a giant bithalamic tumour (Fig. 92B).

3. The Veins

Venous deformations and displacements are described by numerous authors. Their characteristics are reviewed here:

—elevation of the internal cerebral vein in a lateral projection. When the tumour is limited to the posterior thalamus, the posterior third portion of the vein is lifted, becomes rigid or is irregular (Fig. 91).

—when the thalamus as a whole is infiltrated, the internal cerebral vein becomes markedly concave downwards. The lateral deformation of the internal cerebral vein is slight, as long as the tumour is localised in the posterior thalamus. Displacement is all the more important when the tumour extends towards the front. Frontal projections show an elevation of the strio-thalamic veins (Fig. 93).

—compression, absence, deviation towards the midline are the usual displacements of the basal vein in posterior thalamic tumours.

—the presence of thalamic veins in itself is only a cause of suspicion. It is to be associated to other angiographic evidences. These thalamic veins join the internal cerebral vein (Figs. 88 and 93) or the basal vein (Figs. 87, 88 and 93).

—expansions of a thalamic tumour: posterior thalamic tumours are rare. They usually appear as thalamo-peduncular (Figs. 86, 88, 89) or temporo-thalamic masses (Fig. 90). Thus angiographic findings are mixed and comprise the signs of each of the different areas invaded.

Tumours of the Cerebral Peduncles

As in the case of posterior thalamic tumours, peduncular tumours rapidly invade the surrounding areas: the pons and the thalamus. These tumours offer a peculiarity, that is, early occlusion of the aqueduct and its following major result, obstructive hydrocephaly. Pneumoencephalography and pantopaque ventriculography suffice to arrive at a diagnosis (Fig. 95). Angiography, however, is of complementary value in the study of tumoral blood supply.

1. Arteries

a) Frontal Projection of the Posterior Cerebral Artery : the peduncular masses break, deviate or increase the curvature of the peripeduncular segment of the posterior cerebral artery (Figs. 96 and 97). When tumoral localisation is unilateral, the deformation of the posterior cerebral artery permits comparison of the tumoral volume. Global invasion of the peduncles involves a marked increase in curvature of the posterior cerebral arteries.

b) Lateral Projection of the Posterior Cerebral Artery : the lateroperduncular segment of the posterior cerebral artery is rigid or is lowered in a hammock shape, concave upwards (Figs. 97, 98, 99, 100, 101, 106, 108). This deformation may be analagous to a downward temporal herniation. But a frontal projection permits to differentiate a downward temporal herniation from a peduncular tumoral expansion; the former causes a medial deviation, the latter a lateral deviation of the posterior cerebral artery.

Further, a lateral projection shows a rare sign described in 1968 in "Angiographie der Tumoren des Mittelhirnes und seiner Nachbarschaft", in *der Radiologe,* 1968, 11, p. 354–363, namely, kinking of the superior segment of the basilar trunk (Fig. 101).

c) The Posterior Thalamo-perforating Arteries and the Colliculi Quadrigemini and Corporis Callosi Arteries : In cases of unilateral peduncular tumours, a frontal projection permits the viewing of the lateral inclination or deviation of the thalamo-perforating arteries towards the opposite side (Fig. 97).

40

Lateral projections can show the hypertrophy of these arteries, but this does not necessarily entail an invasion of the thalamus. Hypertrophy can also be the result of intracranial hypertension (obstructive hydrocephaly). Deviation and hypertrophy of these arteries leads us to suspect a thalamic expansion of the tumour (Fig. 108).

2. Capillarography

Peduncular tumours, more so than other tumours, are at the origin of a blood stasis in the posterior fossa. In fact, our best capillarographic images of the whole of the posterior fossa were taken in cases of peduncular tumours (Figs. 93, 127 and 128). These often present capillarographic contrasts (Figs. 101, 102 and 103), but the opacities do not represent the whole of the tumour. This technique furnishes a direct addition to vascular topographic information.

3. Veins

Basal Vein. In a lateral projection, dilatation (Fig. 101), dislocation, downward hammock-shaped displacement (Fig. 104), or amputation of the terminal segment of the basal vein is seen. These anomalies of the basal vein are of great diagnostic value. In a frontal projection, external lateral displacement of the basal vein and the lateral mesencephalic vein can be observed.

Lateral Mesencephalic Vein. This vein can be dilated, displaced backwards or often be missing (Figs. 101, 106, 107).

Interpeduncular and Prepontine Veins. These veins are displaced upwards and forwards, or backwards. These displacements involve a deformation of the veins whose characteristic shapes are seen, especially for the prepontine vein, in Figs. 101, 106, 107. When these veins are excluded, a tumoral opacity, cause of the absence, should be looked for (Fig. 103).

The Posterior Mesencephalic Vein. This vein is displaced downward in relation to the basal vein. The dissociation of these two veins (Fig. 105) is direct evidence of peduncular expansion: a sign of the posterior basilo-mesencephalic dissociation.

Extra-Cerebral Tumours Invading the Peduncular Region. Fig. 107 shows the case of a non-operated tumour of the ponto-peduncular region. We report this case to point out the considerable venous displacements. The identification of each vein is possible in this angiography. Fig. 106 illustrates a case of craniopharyngioma with posterior extension. We report this case to point out its venous displacements.

Tumours of the Splenium of the Corpus Callosum

These tumours are not included in the mesencephalon as such. This is the reason why we reproduce the distinctive phlebographic image which points out particular venous displacements as well as circumscribed tumoral opacities (Fig. 110). The region of the splenium can be deformed by tumours in its vicinity, such as internal parietal tumours.

Ependymoma of the IIIrd Ventricle

We report here the case of an ependymoma that involves the IIIrd ventricle. Fig. 111 shows venous displacements, hypertrophy of the ventricular veins and tumoral capillarography. Note, for the sake of comparison, a normal angiography of the ventricular veins (Fig. 69).

Meningiomas of the Tentorium

In pneumoencephalography, meningiomas of the tentorium appear as expansive masses in the mesencephalic area. Angiography permits to define the nature of the tumour in a great majority of cases. These tumours always grow considerably before causing symptoms. Their important mass is responsible for the displacement of the calcified pineal body, as shown in Fig. 112, as well as the pathological spread of the posterior cerebral arteries, seen frontally in Fig. 113. The meningial arteries of the internal intra-cranial carotid arteries (Bernasconi) are often very enlarged in cases of meningiomas of the tentorium (Figs. 113, 114, 115 and 118), as is the occipital artery (branch of the external carotid). In one of our cases, we found a hammock sign (Fig. 116) similar in shape to certain pinealomas (Fig. 81). In the case of a meningioma, however, the hammock is accompanied by an important enlargement of the distance between the posterior cerebral arteries. Capillarography or tumoral opacification of the venous phase often permits to outline a great part of the tumoral mass.
Medial meningiomas dislocate, embody and displace the posterior pericallosal and posterior choroidal arteries. These arterial displacements, however, follow a forward direction opposite to that taken by pineal and thalamic tumours. In certain rare cases, the origin of the tumour is doubtful when a thalamic tumour has embodied the posterior choroidal arteries. Other indications will be of help in finding the origin of the tumour. A characteristic sign of a meningioma of the free edge

of the tentorium is the dissociation of the posterior cerebral artery and the postero-superior cerebellar artery in frontal (Fig. 118) and lateral (Fig. 119) projections. The displacement of these arteries is divergent, due to the expansion of the meningioma situated between them.

Phlebograms are greatly dislocated by these voluminous meningial tumours. The example given in Fig. 119 shows important disturbances in arterial topography, marked tumoral capillarography, as well as important venous displacements.

Aneurysms of the Mesencephalic Area

When aneurysms cause hematomas, they provoke arterial and venous displacements. These signs are useful in angiographic diagnosis, as seen in Fig. 120. An abnormal capillarography may be visible in the region of the hematoma (Fig. 121).

Arterio-venous Aneurysms

Arterio-venous aneurysms are reported in order to complete the angiographic picture of this region. These frequent malformations can follow the topography of mesencephalic arteries (Fig. 122) or produce enormous dilatations of the basal vein (Fig. 123).

Mesencephalic Angiography in Active Hydrocephaly

1. The arteries of the mesencephalon, which are generally faint in a normal angiogram, appear much more sharply in the case of important non-tumoral active hydrocephaly. This improved visibility of the mesencephalic arteries is sufficiently pronounced to attract attention. A partial segmentary rigidity is also apparent. Such active hydrocephaly entails very good visibility of the choroidal arteries in a frontal view (Fig. 124).

An indication of significance of such a ventricular dilatation is the crossing of the medial posterior choroidal arteries with the postero-lateral choroidal arteries. The former is, in effect, markedly displaced backwards because of its close connection with the posterior wall of the dilated IIIrd ventricle. On the other hand, the postero-lateral choroidal artery is only slightly displaced. This phenomenon is illustrated in Fig. 125. In carotid angiography, hydrocephaly shows an increase in curvature of the anterior pericallosal artery, much the same as the posterior pericallosal artery, whose curvature is also increased by ventricular dilatation.

2. The Veins (Fig. 126). The basal vein is displaced backwards and downwards, so much so that its angulation in a frontal view is blunted. The other mesencephalic veins undergo variable displacements or no displacement. We have observed a slight elevation of the lateral mesencephalic and pre-central veins through dilatation of the IVth ventricle. Finally, the internal cerebral vein is lowered and displaced slightly backwards. The superior thalamic vein can be dilated. The lateral ventricular veins are displaced from the midline to the exterior.

Angiographic anomalies are generally dependent on a topographic type of hydrocephaly up to a certain stage of ventricular dilatation. Consequently, vascular deformations in the mesencephalic region depend on the orientation of the predominant pressure.

3. Capillarography. Increased intracranial pressure in active hydrocephaly, especially when caused by a mesencephalic tumour, induces a main stasis in the posterior fossa so that it becomes possible to produce strongly contrasted pictures (Fig. 93, 127, 128).

References

Abrams, H. L.: Angiography, Boston: Little Brown & Co 1961.

Bernasconi,V., Cassinari,V.: Un segno carotidografico tipico di meningioma del tentorio. Chirurgia **11**, 586–588 (1956).

Bradac, G. B., Wackenheim, A., Braun, J. P.: Contribution à l'étude du phlébogramme de l'angiographie vertébrale. Neurochirurgia **12** (I), 1–16 (1969).

Braun, J. P.: Les veines cérébrales. France méd. No 7, 317–325 (1967).

— Wackenheim, A.: Capillarographie cérébrale. J. Radiol. Électrol. **50**, 532 (1969).

— — Capillarographie cérébrale. Neurochirurgia **12** (3), 94–99 (1969).

Bray, P. F., Carter, S., Taveras, J. M.: Brainstem tumors in children. Neurology (Minneap.) **8**, 1 (1958).

Bull, J. W. D.: The volume of the cerebral ventricles. Neurology (Minneap.) **11**, 1 (1961).

Carpenter, M. B., Noback, C. R., Moss, M. L.: The anterior choroidal artery. Its origins, course, distribution and variations. Arch. Neurol. Psychiat. (Chic.) **71**, 714 (1954).

Castellanos, F., Ruggiero, G.: Meningiomas of the posterior fossa. Acta radiol. (Stockh.), Suppl. 104, 1 vol. (1953).

Chase, N. E., Taveras, J. M.: Cerebral angiography in the diagnosis of suprasellar tumors. Amer. J. Roentgenol. **84**, 154 (1961).

Columella, F., Papo, T.: Vertebral angiography in supra-tentorial expansive processuses. Acta radiol. (Stockh.) **46**, 178 (1956).

Cummins, F. M., Taveras, J. M., Schlesinger, E. B.: Treatment of gliomas of the third ventricle and pinealomas; with special reference to the value of radiotherapy. Neurology (Minneap.) **10**, 1031 (1960).

Cushing, H.: The pituitary body and its disorders. Philadelphia: J. B. Lippincott Company 1912.

David, M., Bernard-Weill, E., Dilenge, D.: Les tumeurs de la glande pinéale. Ann. Endocr. (Paris) **24**, 287–330 (1963).

Decker, K. (ed.): Klinische Neuroradiologie. Stuttgart: Thieme 1960.

— Backmund: Angiographie des Hirnkreislaufs. 1 vol. Stuttgart: Thieme 1968.

Dilenge, D., David, M.: L'opacification des artères thalamique au cours de l'angiographie vertébrale. Neurochirurgie **11**, 511–518 (1965).

Djindjian, R., Bories, J.: Principes généraux du diagnostic des processus expansifs intra-crâniens par l'angiographie vertébrale. In: Diagnostico neuroradiologico (Solé Llénas et Wackenheim), Toray, ed., 1 vol., p. 343–352. Barcelona 19...

Economos, D., Prosalentis: L'artère cérébelleuse supérieure dans les tumeurs de la fosse postérieure. Acta radiol. (Stockh.) 267–277 (1963).

Frugoni, P., Nori, A., Galligioni, F., Giammusso, V.: A particular angiographic sign in meningiomas of the tentorium: the artery of Bernasconi and Cassinari. Neurochirurgia **2**, 142–152 (1959).

— — — — A particular angiographic sign in meningiomas of the tentorium: The artery of Bernasconi and Cassinari. Neurochirurgia **2**, 142 (1960).

Galloway, J. R., Greitz, T.: The medial and lateral choroid arteries. An anatomic and roentgenographic study. Acta radiol. (Stockh.) **53**, 353–366 (1960).

References

Gladstone, R. J., Wakeley, C. P. G.: The pineal organ, p. 467. London: Baillière, Tindall & Cox 1940.

Hara, K., Fujino: Thalamoperforate artery. Acta radiol. (Stockh.) **5**, 192–200 (1966).

Huang, Y. P., Wolf, B. S.: Precentral cerebellar vein in angiography. Acta radiol. (Diag.) (Stockh.) **5**, 250–262 (1966).

— — Veins of the posterior fossa—superior or Galenic draining group. Amer. J. Roentgenol. **95**, 808–821 (1965).

— — The vein of the lateral recess of the fourth ventricle and its tributaries—Roentgen appearance and anatomic relationships. Amer. J. Roentgenol. **101**, 1–21 (1967).

— — Angiographic features of fourth ventricle tumors with special reference to the posterior inferior cerebellar artery. Amer. J. Roentgenol. **107**, 543–564 (1969).

— — Angiographic features of brain stem tumors and differential diagnosis from fourth ventricle tumors. Amer. J. Roentgenol. (Accepted for publication).

— — Antin, S. P., Okudera, T.: The veins of the posterior fossa—anterior or petrosal draining group. Amer. J. Roentgenol. **104**, 36–56 (1968).

— — — — Kim, I. H.: Angiographic features of aqueductal stenosis. Amer. J. Roentgenol. **104**, 90–108 (1968).

Isfort, A.: Spontane Hirnblutungen. 1 vol. Berlin: Schering A.G. 1967.

Johanson, C.: The central veins and deep dural sinuses of the brain. Acta radiol. (Stockh.), Suppl. 107 (1954).

Kitay, J. I., Altschule, M. D.: The pineal gland. A review of the physiologic literature, p. vii. Cambridge, Massachusetts: Harvard University Press 1954.

Krayenbühl, H., Richter, H. R.: Die zerebrale Angiographie, 1. Aufl. Stuttgart: Thieme 1952.

— Yasargil, M. G.: Die vaskulären Erkrankungen im Gebiet der Arteria Vertebralis and Arteria Basialis. Stuttgart: Thieme 1957.

— — Die zerebrale Angiographie. 1 vol. Stuttgart: Georg Thieme 1965.

Kundert, J. G.: Pinealom und Tumoren des III. Ventrikels. Diss. Zürich 1963.

Laine, E., Delandtsheer, J. M., Galibert, P., Delandtsheer-Arnott, G.: Phlebography in tumors of the hemispheres and central grey matter. Acta radiol. (Stockh.) **46**, 203 (1956).

Lazorthes, G.: Vascularisation et circulation cérébrales. I vol. Masson & Cie. 1961.

Lefebvre, J. C., Faure, C., Salomon, G.: Etude radiologique des gliomes infiltrants du tronc cérébral. Acta radiol. (Stockh.) **1**, 343–357 (1963).

Lin, P. M., Mokrohisky, J. F., Stauffer, J. M., Scott, M.: The importance of the deep cerebral veins in deep cerebral angiography. J. Neurosurg. **12**, 256 (1955).

Lindgren, E.: Percutaneous angiography of the vertebral artery. Acta radiol. (Stockh.) **33**, 389 (1950).

Löfgren, F. O.: Vertebral angiography in the diagnosis of tumors in the pineal region. Acta radiol. (Stockh.) **60**, 108–124 (1958).

Lysholm, E., Ebenius, B., Sahlstedt, H.: Das Ventrikulogram. Teil III. Dritter und vierter Ventrikel. Acta radiol. (Stockh.), Suppl. **26**, 124 (1935).

Maslowski, H. A.: Vertebral angiography. Percutaneous lateral atlanto-Occipital method. Brit. J. Surg. **43**, 1 (1955).

Mones, R.: Vertebral angiography. An analysis of 106 cases. Radiology **76**, 230 (1961).

Namin, P.: L'angiographie vertebrale. Paris: Doin et Cie. 1955.

North, P.: Nystagmus on clonus retractorius. Thèse de médecine No 11, Strasbourg 1967.

Padget, D. H.: Development of cranial venous system in man, from viewpoint of comparative anatomy. Carnegie Inst. Publ. 611, Contrib. Emb. 36, 79–140 (1957).

Pernkopf, E.: Topographische Anatomie des Menschen. 1 vol. München-Berlin: Urban & Schwarzenberg 1960.

Potts, D. G., Taveras, J. M.: Differential Diagnosis of Space-occupying lesions in the region of the thalamus by cerebral angiography. Acta radiol. (Stockh.) 1, 373–384 (1963).

Pribram, H. F. W.: Angiographic appearances in acute intracranial hypertension. Neurology (Minneap.) 11, 10 (1961).

Radner, S.: Vertebral angiography by catheterization. A new method employed in 221 cases. Acta radiol. (Stockh.) Suppl. 87 (1951).

Rauber-Kopsch, F.: Lehrbuch der Anatomie des Menschen, Bd. II. Leipzig: G. Thieme 1948.

Richter, H. S. R.: Phlebogram in brainstem tumors. Acta radiol. (Stockh.) 40, 182–187 (1953).

Ring, B. A.: Variations in the striate and other cerebral veins affecting measurements of the venous angle. Acta radiol. (Stockh.) 52, 433 (1959).

Ruggiero, G., Dettori, P.: La soustraction d'image en angiographie cérébrale bidirectionnelle simultanée. 1 vol. Neuchatel (Suisse): Delachaux et Niestle.

Sheldon, P.: A special needle for percutaneous vertebral angiography. Brit. J. Radiol. 29, 231 (1956).

Sjögren, S. E.: Percutaneous vertebral angiography. Acta radiol. (Stockh.) 40, 113 (1953).

Sugar, O., Holden, L. B., Powell, C. B.: Vertebral angiography. Amer. J. Roentgenol. 61, 166 (1949).

Sutton, D.: Radiologic aspects of pontine gliomata. Acta radiol. (Stockh.) 40, 234 (1953).

Taveras, S. M., Wood, E. H.: Diagnostic Neuroradiology. Baltimore: Williams & Wilkins Co. 1964.

Thevenot, C.: Les artères du système nerveux central. 1 vol. Vigot Frères 1959.

Tovi, D., Schisano, G., Liliequist, B.: Primary tumors of the region of the thalamus. J. Neurosurg. 18, 730–740 (1961).

Viale, G. L., Rosa, M.: Studio angiografico del sistema venoso vertebro-basilare. Sistema Nervoso-Longanesi, Milano 1968:
(I) Le vene ponto-mesencephaliche 3, 131–142.
(II) La vena sopraculminara (vermiana superiore) 3, 143–146.
(III) La vena vermiana inferiore, 4, 280–285.
(IV) La vena cerebellare precentrale, 4, 286–294.
(V) La vena cerebellare marginale, 5, 1—4.
(VI) La vena cerebellare antero-superiore, 5, 1—6.
(VII) Le vene cerebellari emisferiche, 5, 1—6.

Wackenheim, A., Braun, J. P., Bradac, G. B.: Angiographie der Tumoren des Mittelhirnes und seiner Nachbarschaft. Radiologe 8 (II), 354–363 (1968).

Westberg, G.: The arteries of cerebral ganglia. VII. Symposium Neuroradiologicum, 1964, New York, p. 32.

— Arteries of the basal ganglia. Acta radiol. (Stockh.) 581—596 (1966).

Wolf, B. S., Huang, Y. P.: The subependymal veins of the lateral ventricles. Amer. J. Roentgenol. 91, 406–426 (1964).

— — Newman, C. M.: The lateral anastomotic mesencephalic vein and other variations in drainage of the basal cerebral vein. Amer. J. Roentgenol. 89, 411–422 (1963).

— Newman, C. M., Schlesinger, B.: Diagnostic value of the deep cerebral veins in cerebral angiography. Radiology 64, 161 (1955).

References

Yasargil, M. G.: Die Vertebralisangiographie; ihre Bedeutung für die Diagnose der Tumoren. Acta neurochir. (Wien), Suppl. **9**, 1–108 (1962).
Zatz, L. M., Hanberg, J. W., Gifford, D., Belza, J.: The diagnosis of tumors of the splenium of the corpus callosum. Amer. J. Roentgenol. **101**, 130–140 (1967).
Ziedses des Plantes, B. G.: Planigraphie en subtractie. Röntgenographische Differentiatiemethoden. Thesis, 1934.
— Subtraktion. Eine röntgenographische Methode zur separaten Abbildung bestimmter Teile des Objekts. Fortschr. Röntgenstr. **52**, 69 (1935).

Illustrations

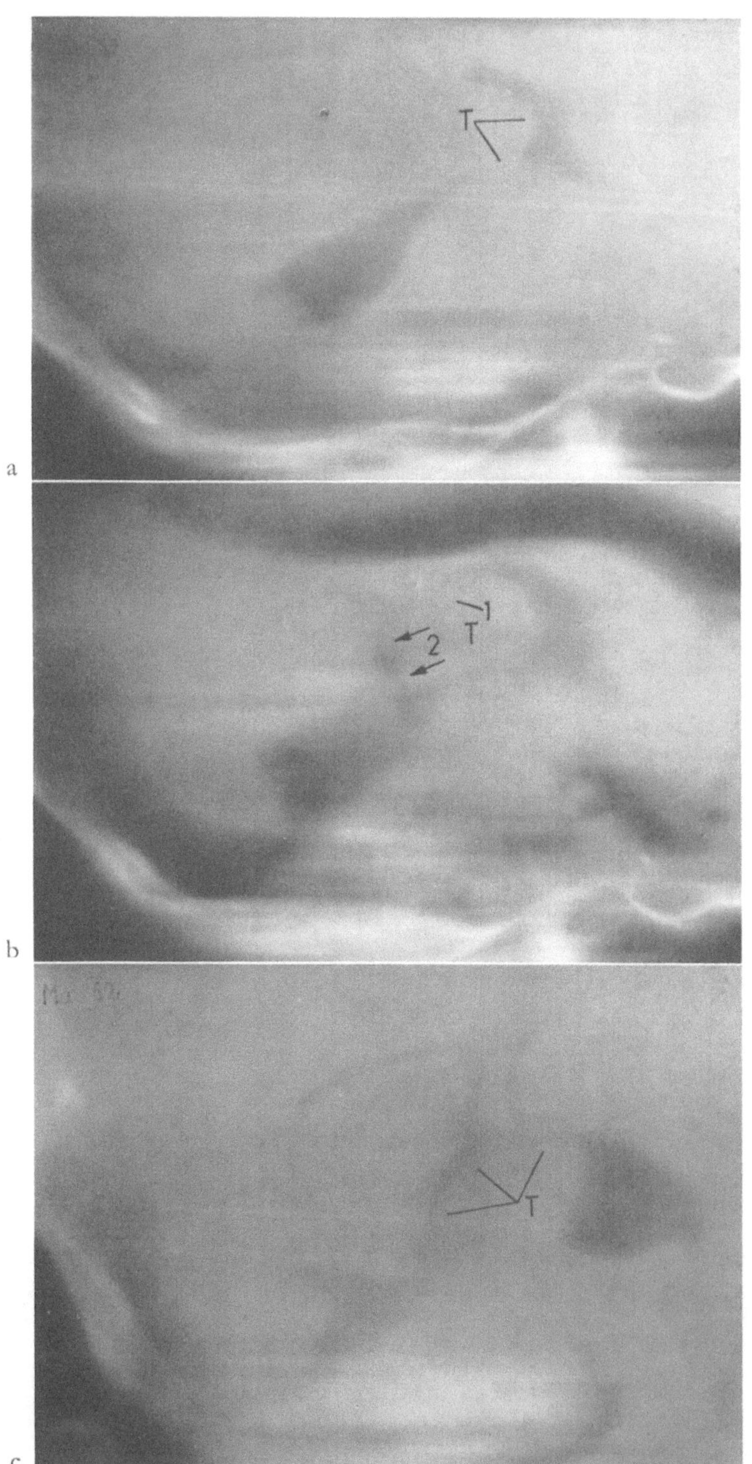

Fig. 1 a–f
Medial pneumostratigraphy in
6 cases of pineal area tumours.
a) Marked concavity of the
posterior wall of the IIIrd ventricle due to tumoral compression. The aqueduct of Sylvius
is narrowed and elongated.
b) Anomalies of "a" are sup-
plemented by: backward displacement of the ambient cistern; displacement and enlargement of the prevermian cistern.
c) The quadrigeminal cistern
outlines the superior contours
of the tumour.

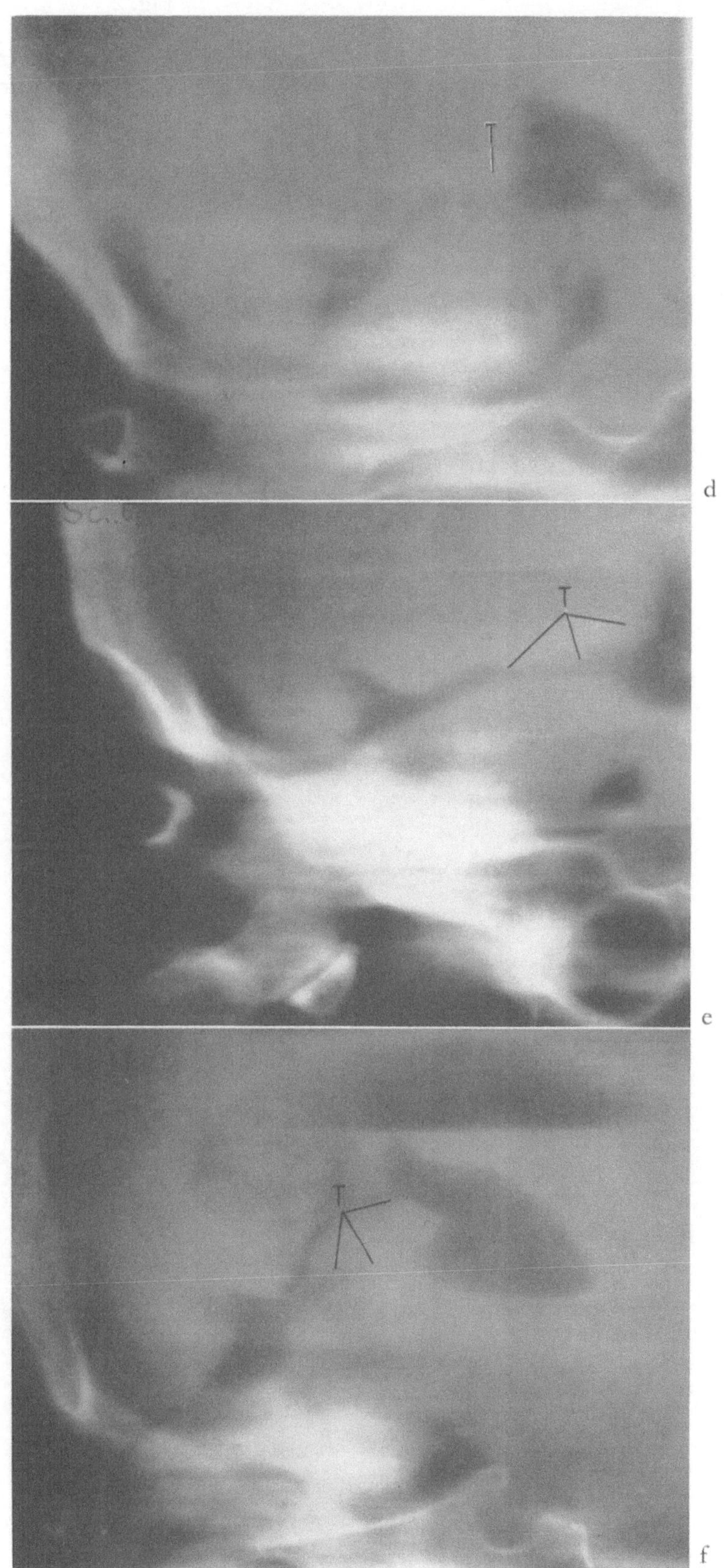

d) Enlargement and angulation of the aqueduct by the lower pole of the tumour.

e) These anomalies are more accentuated in this case than in "d".

f) Tumoral expansion bears principally downwards and backwards. The posterior wall of the IIIrd ventricle suffers no alteration

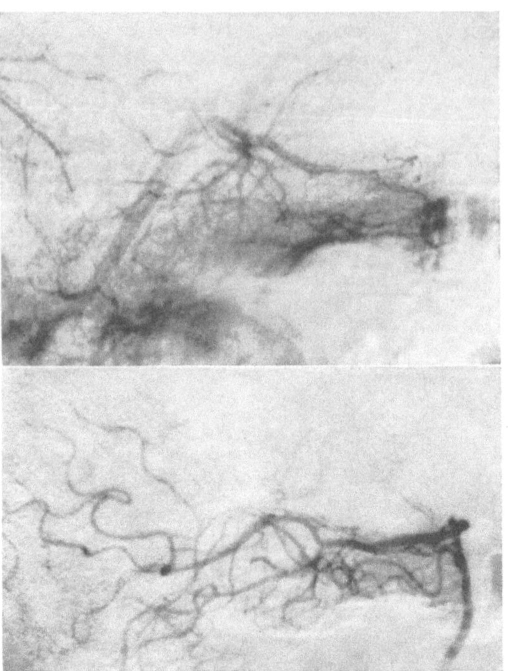

Fig. 2
Normal lateral phlebogram (above) and arteriogram (below) of the mesencephalic region. The posterior portion of the internal cerebral vein alone is opacified by vertebral angiography

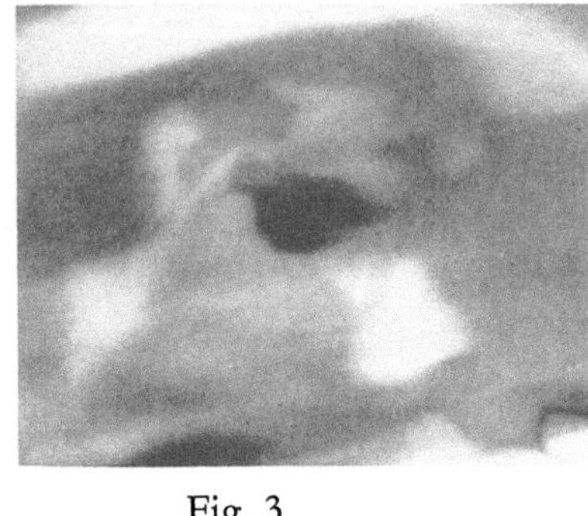

Fig. 3
Important peduncular calcification (non operated) evidenced through medial sagittal pneumostratigraphy

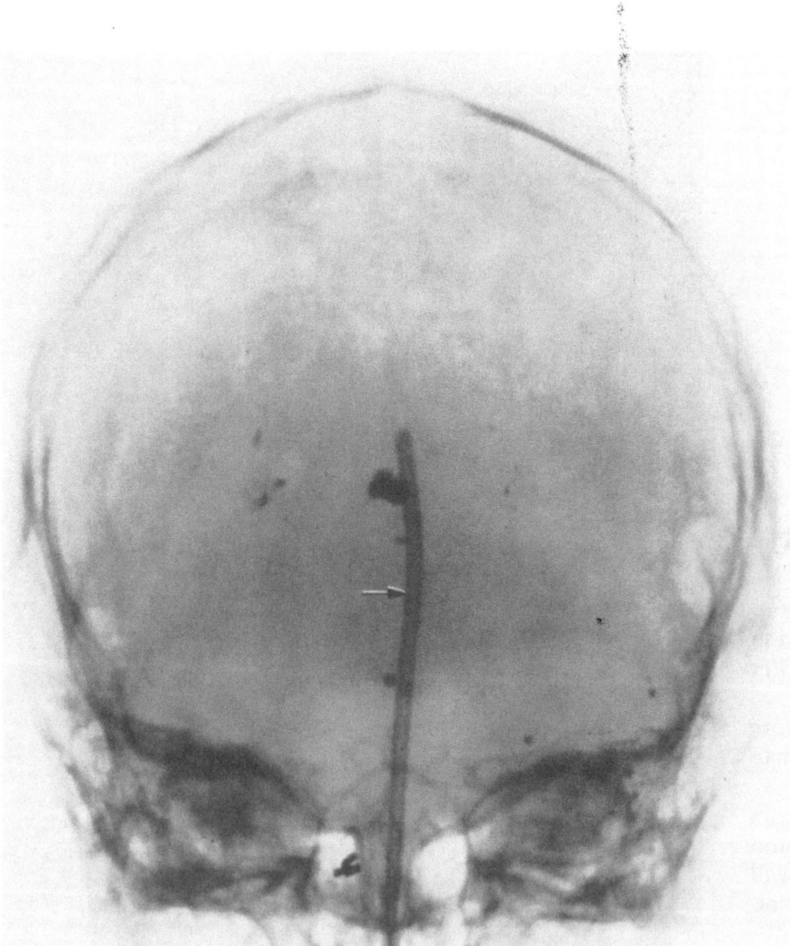

Fig. 4
Glioma of the right cerebral peduncle; displaced drain in the aqueduct of Sylvius. The angulation of this opaque drain indicates the tumoral expansion and permits to follow its evolution

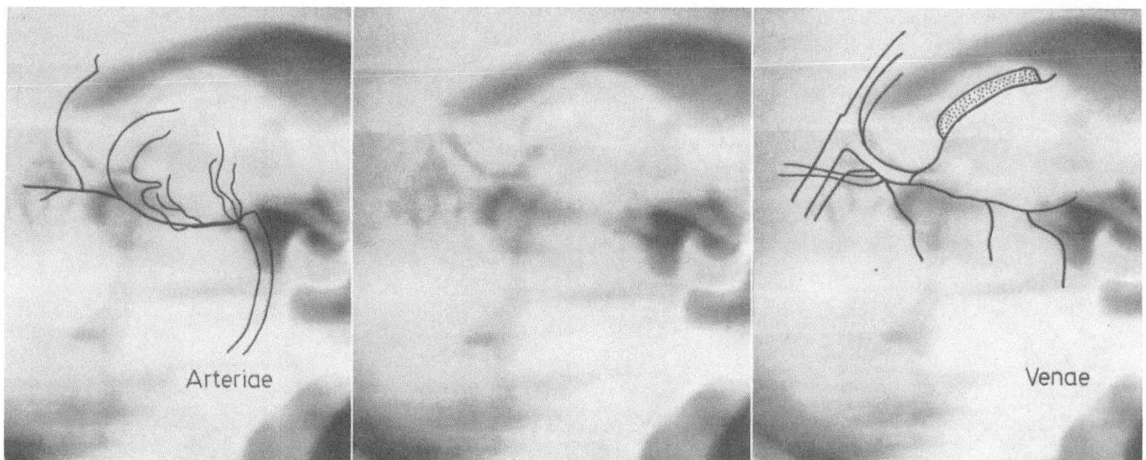

Fig. 5. Drawing of the arteries and veins on a medial sagittal pneumo-stratigram showing the relation between these vessels and the ventriculo-cisternal cavities in profile

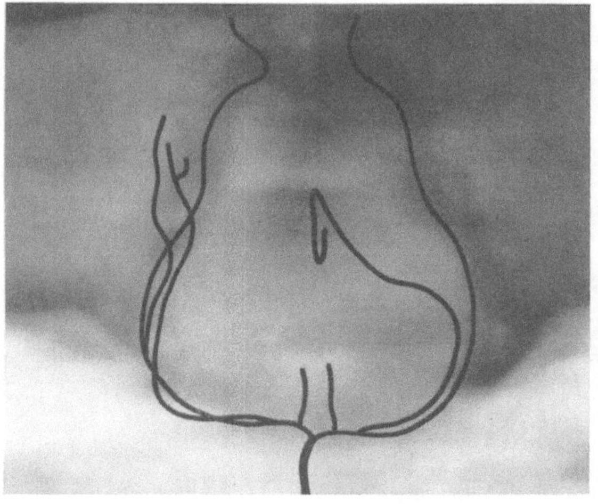

Fig. 6. Drawing of the arteries and veins in frontal pneumo-stratigraphy of the cerebral trunk

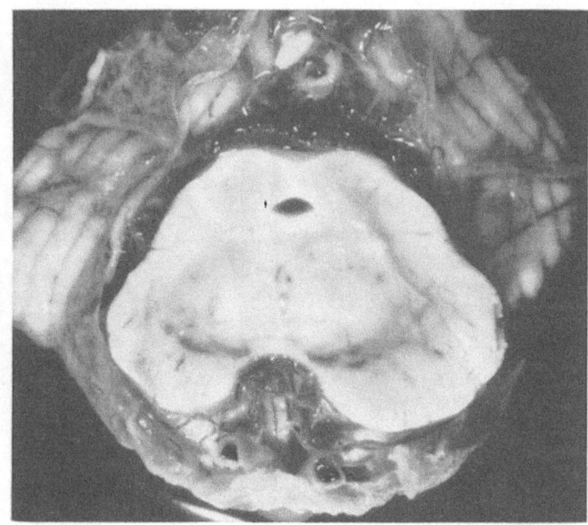

Fig. 7. The cerebral peduncles can be unequal in size especially in atrophic after-effects of circulatory origin

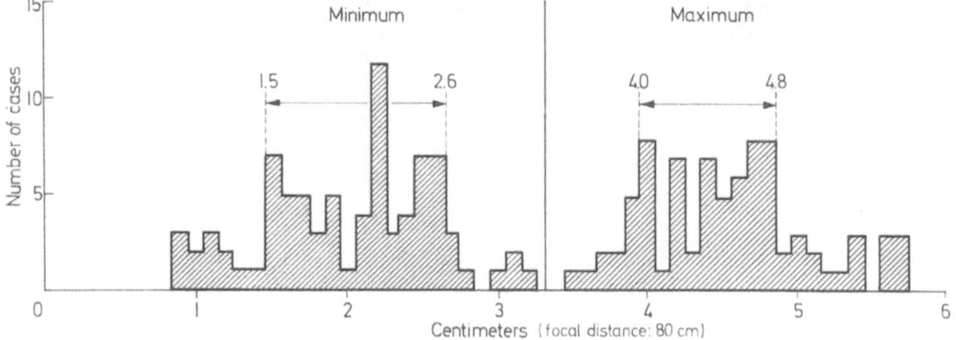

Fig. 8. In a frontal view the minimum distance between the posterior cerebral arteries is 15 to 25 mms near the tentorium. The maximum distance in a frontal view between the posterior cerebral arteries is generally 40 to 50 mms at the level of the latero-peduncular segment

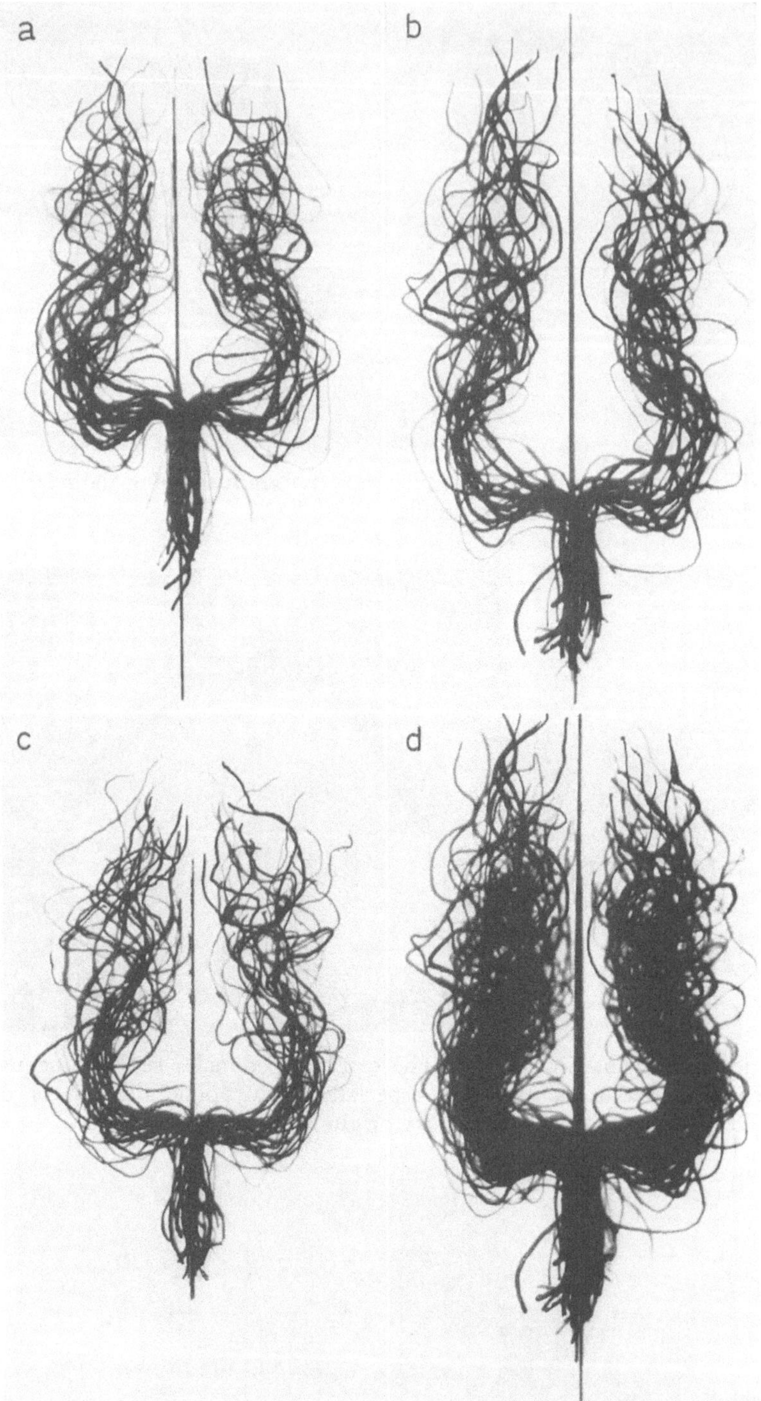

Fig. 9a–d
Tracings of angiographic frontal views of posterior cerebral arteries
in 90 normal non-selected cases. a, b, c) Superposition of 30 different
cases. d) Summation of the 90 cases

Fig. 10
The angle formed in a lateral view by the posterior cerebral artery and the basilar trunk is variable, as seen in the superposition of 90 normal cases

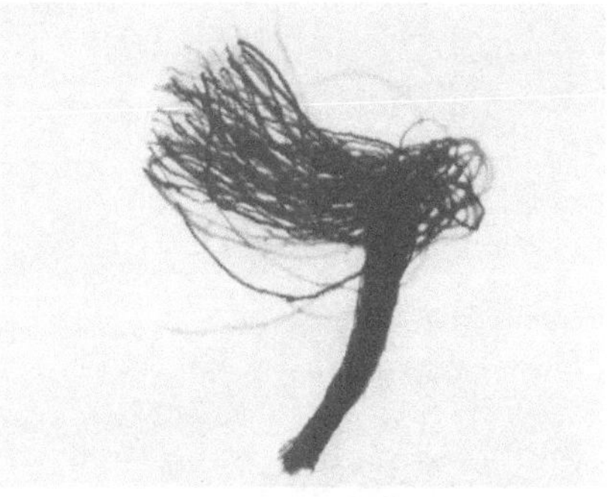

Fig. 11
Different types of posterior thalamo-perforating arteries in a frontal view

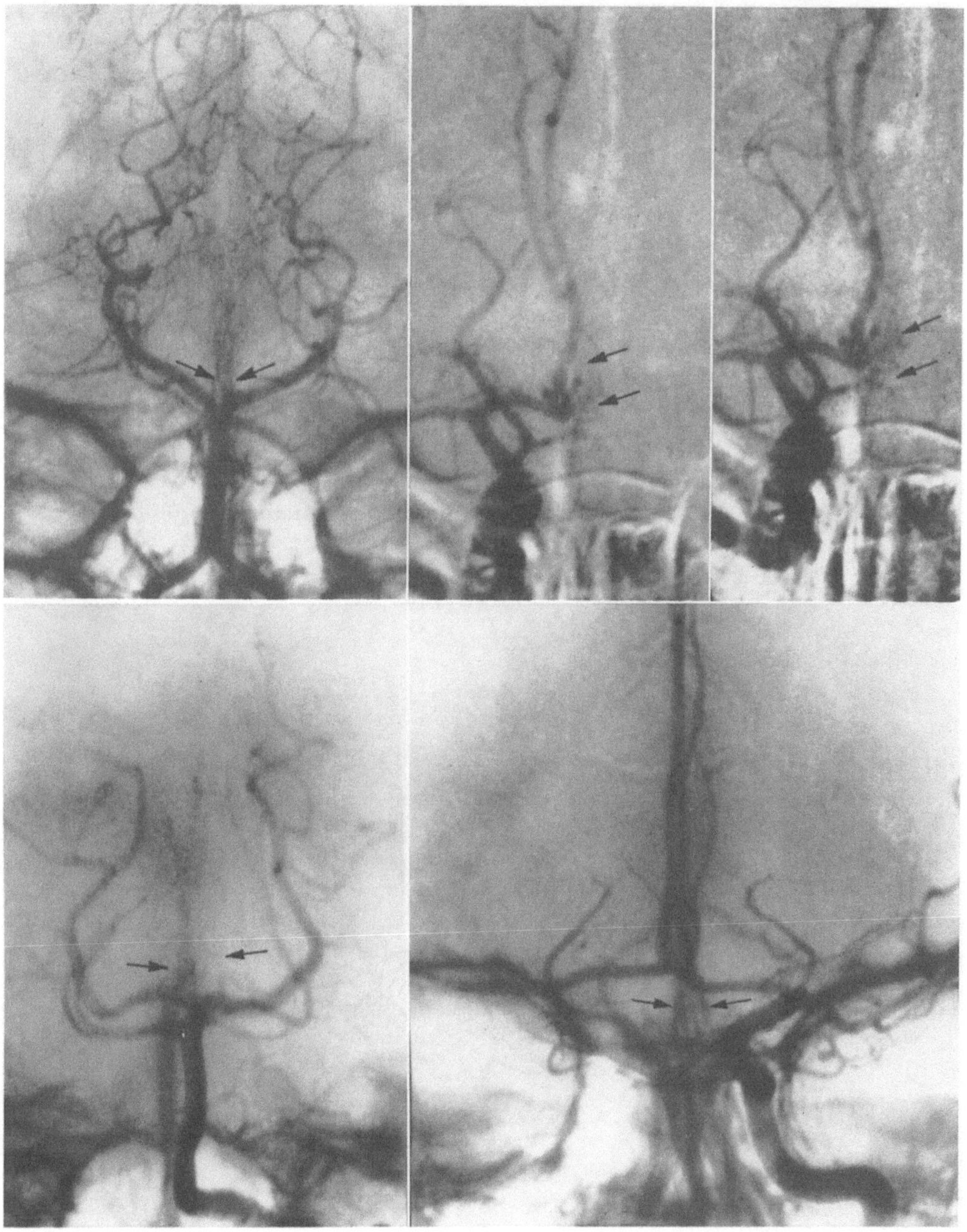

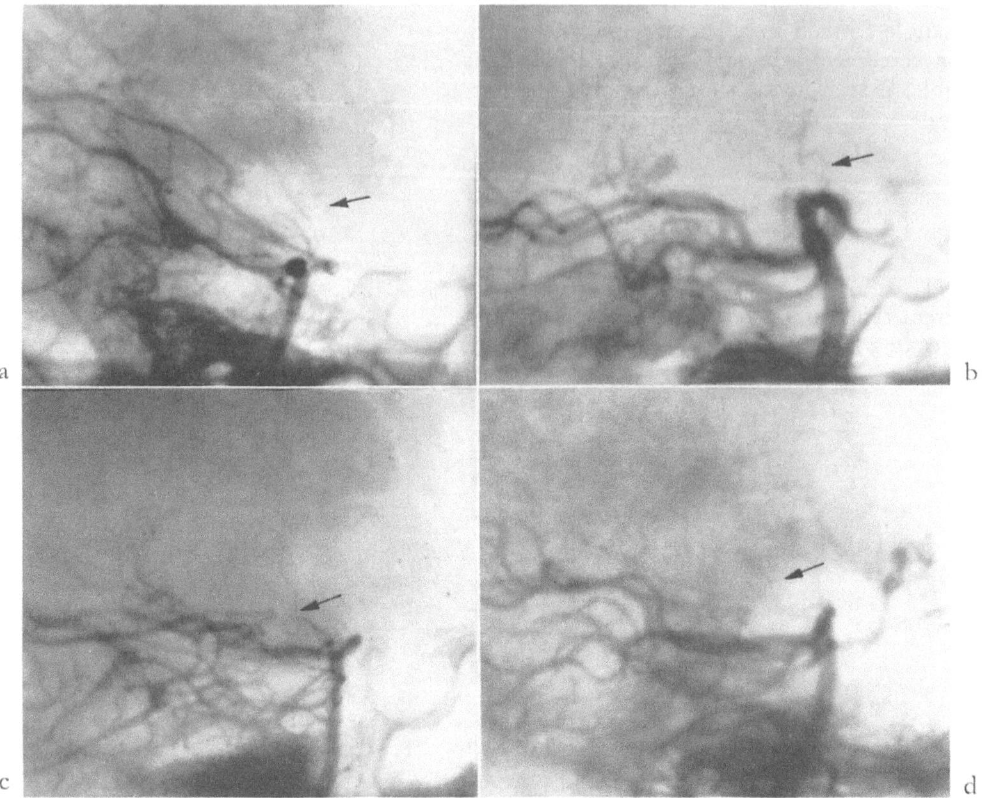

Fig. 12a–d
Different types of thalamo-perforating arteries in a lateral view. a) Anterior thalamo-perforating arteries. b, c, d) Posterior thalamo-perforating arteries

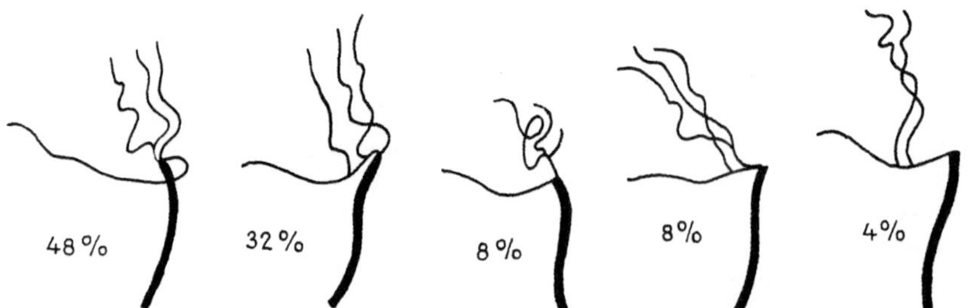

Fig. 13
Arteriae thalamo-perforatae posteriores

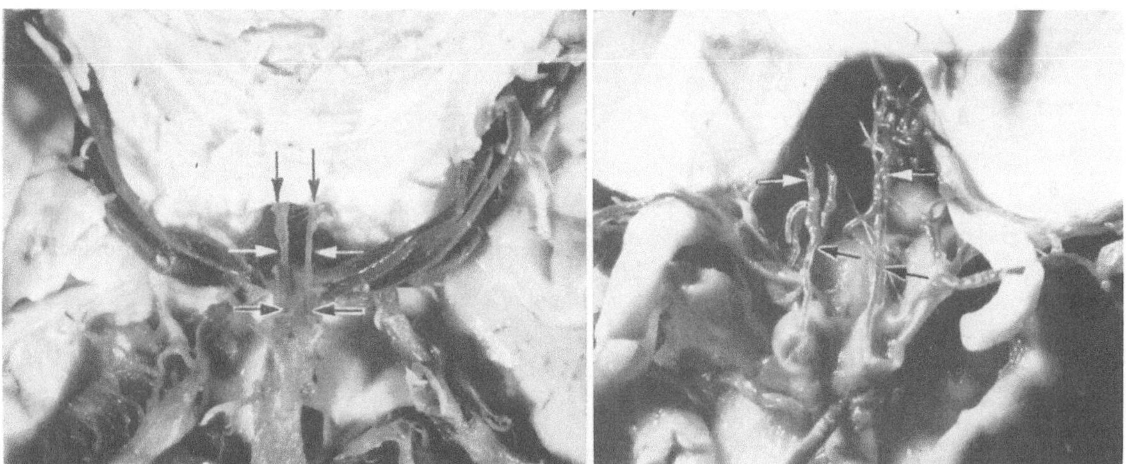

Fig. 14. The posterior thalamo-perforating arteries leave the basilar trunk near the point of departure of the posterior cerebral arteries. Upon dissection it can be observed that their calibre is heavy compared to the view in angiography

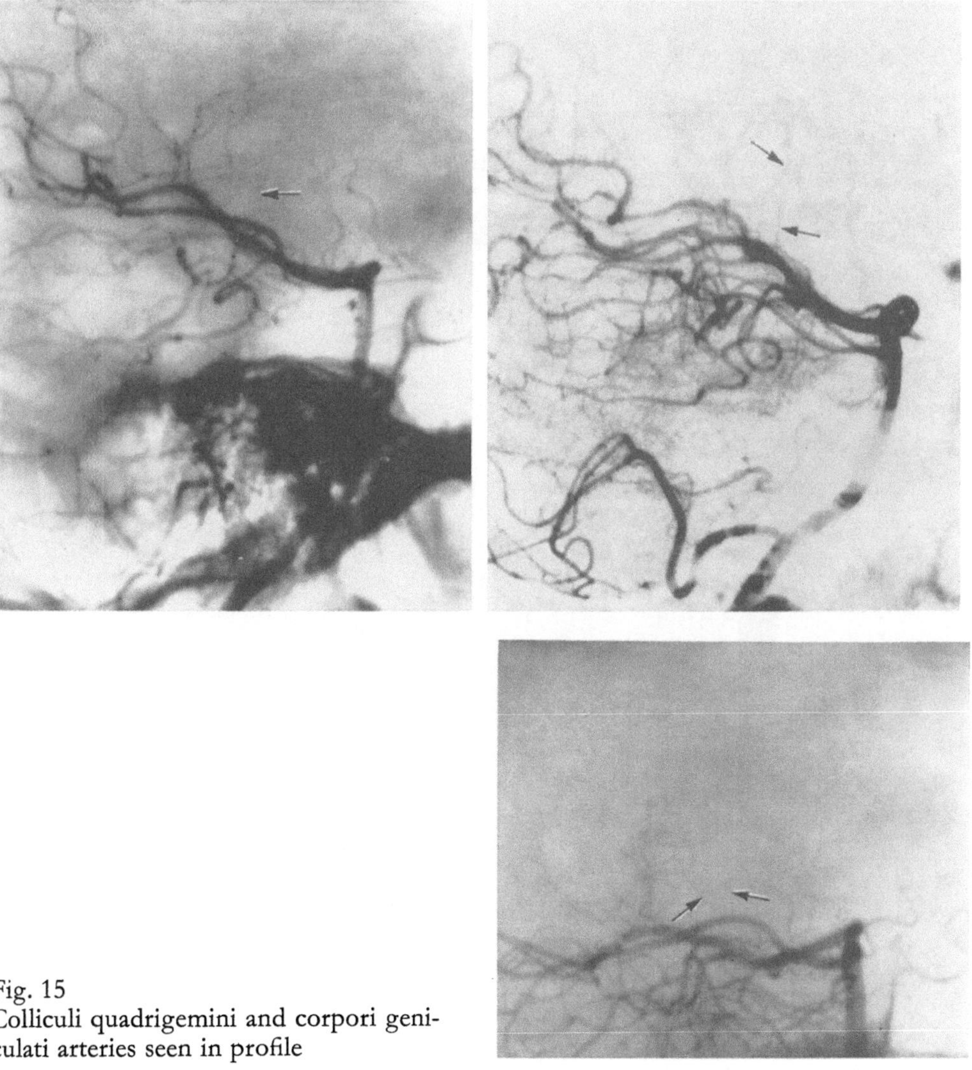

Fig. 15
Colliculi quadrigemini and corpori geniculati arteries seen in profile

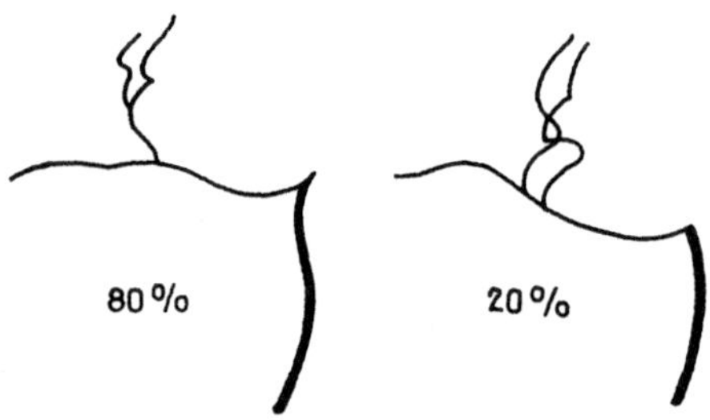

Fig. 16
Arteriae colliculi quadrigemini et corpori geniculati

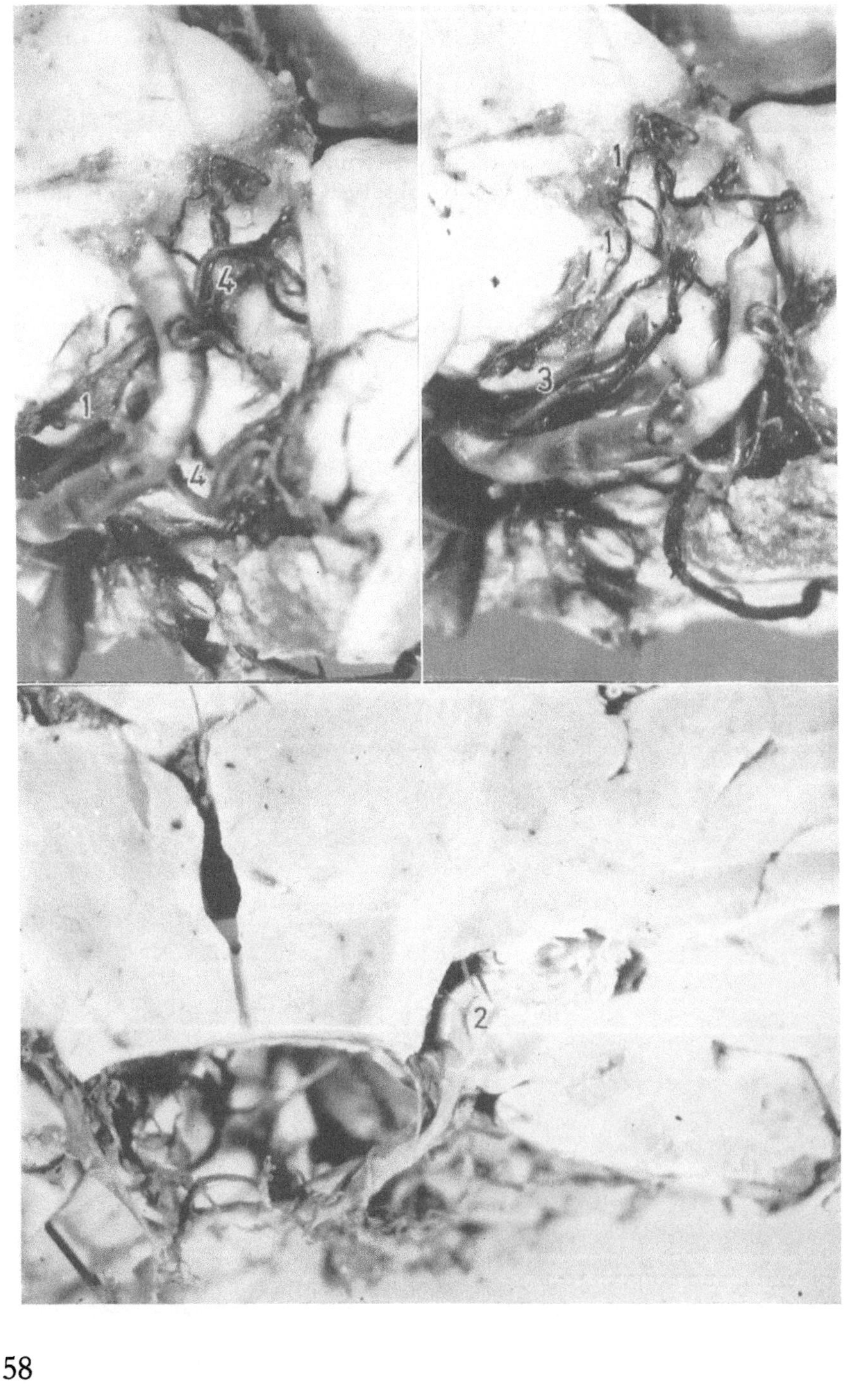

Fig. 17
Dissection of the arteries. *1* Colliculi quadrigemini artery. *2* Corpori geniculati artery. *3* Postero-medial choroidal artery. *4* Postero-lateral choroidal artery

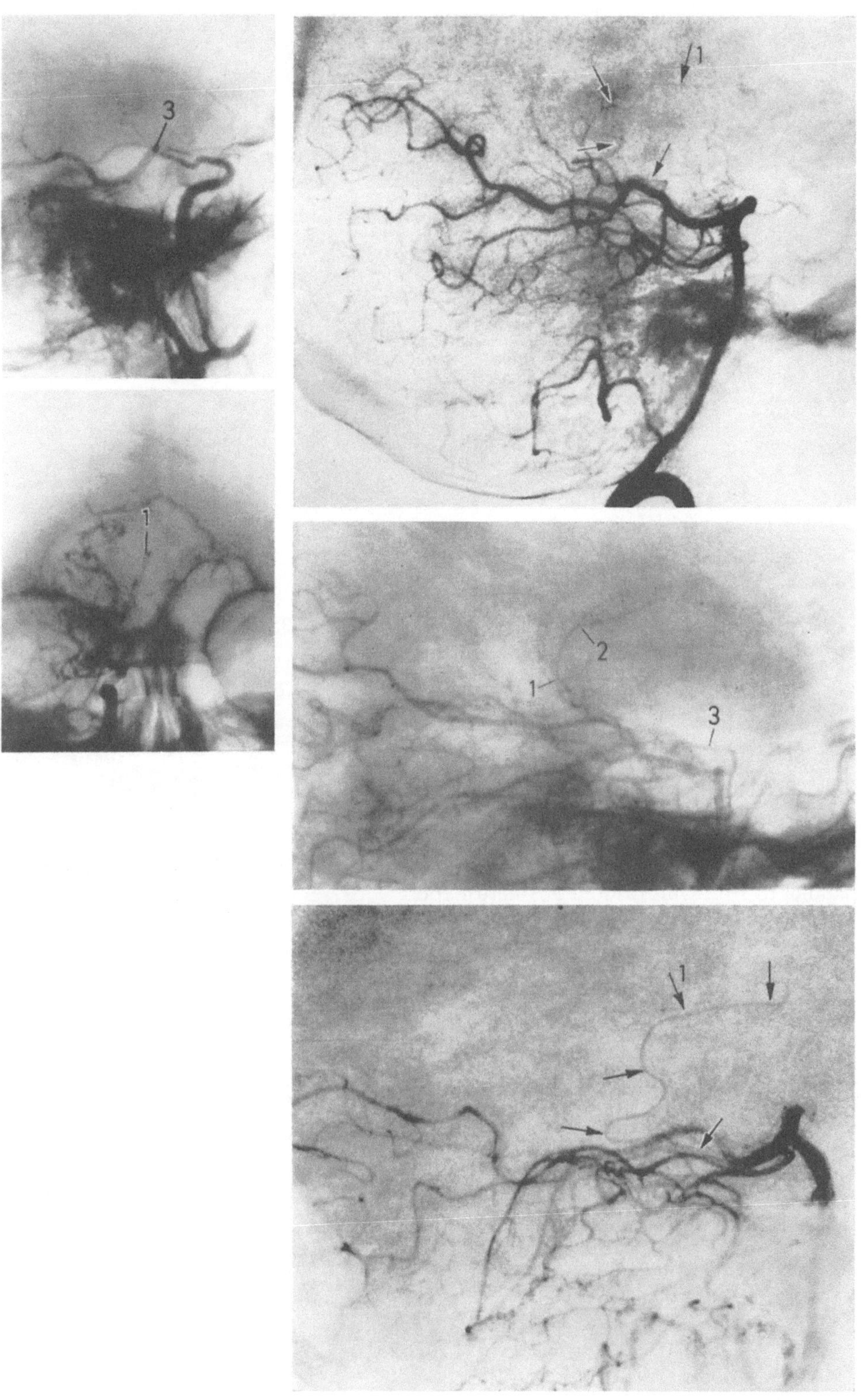

Fig. 18. Postero-medial choroidal artery (*1*) having two terminal branches (*2*). Note the departure of this artery (*3*) near the basilar trunk

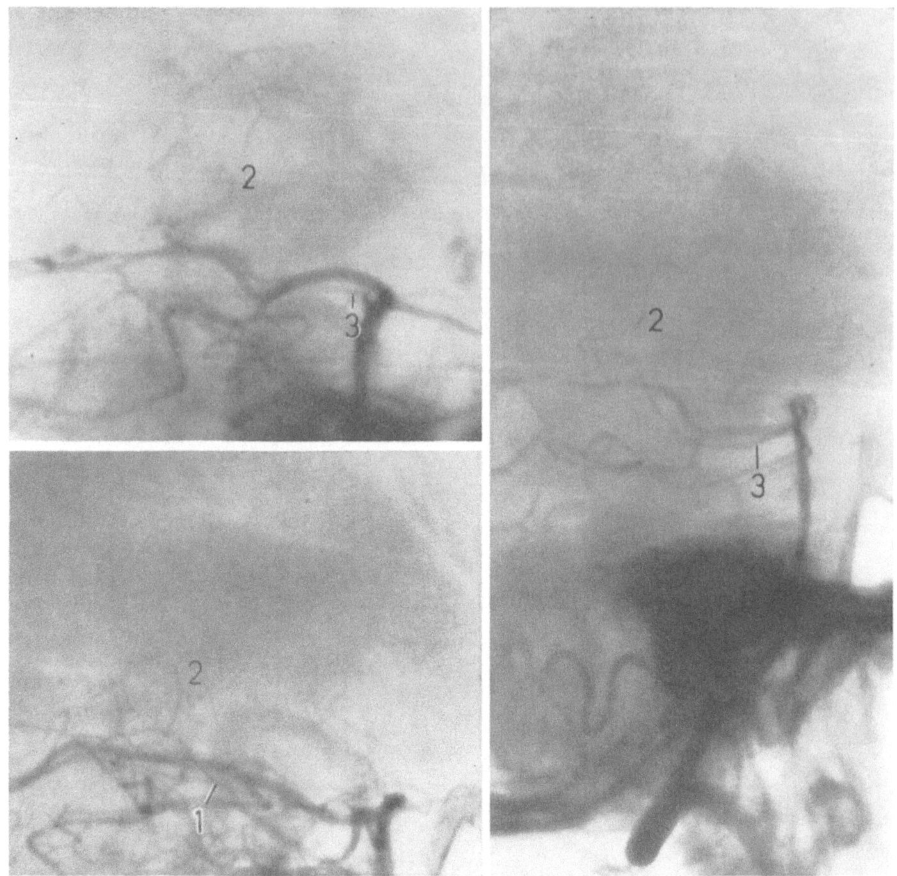

Fig. 19
Postero-medial choroidal artery. *1* Postero-medial choroidal artery courses parallel to P2. *2* Bifurcation. *3* Anterior root

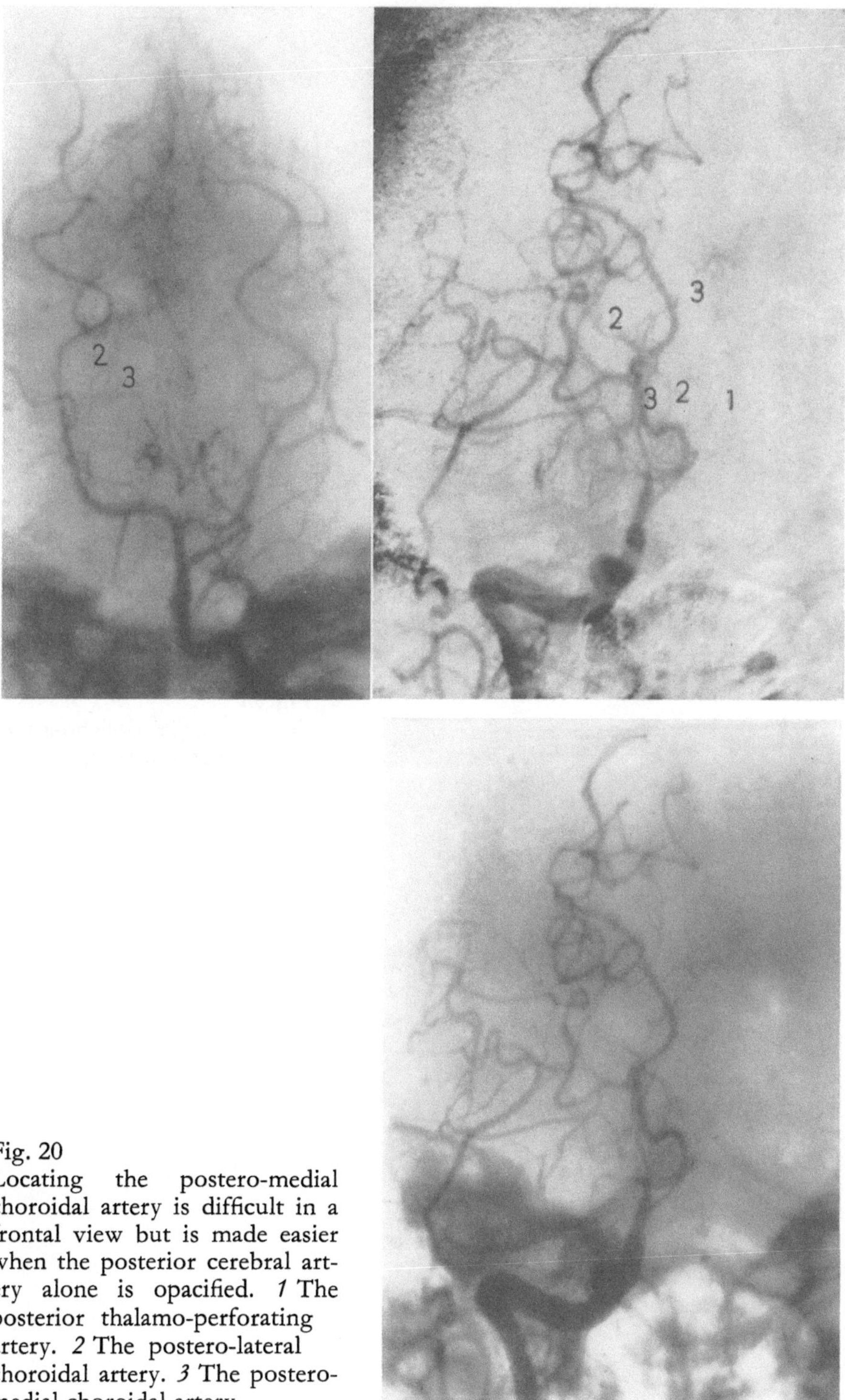

Fig. 20
Locating the postero-medial choroidal artery is difficult in a frontal view but is made easier when the posterior cerebral artery alone is opacified. *1* The posterior thalamo-perforating artery. *2* The postero-lateral choroidal artery. *3* The postero-medial choroidal artery

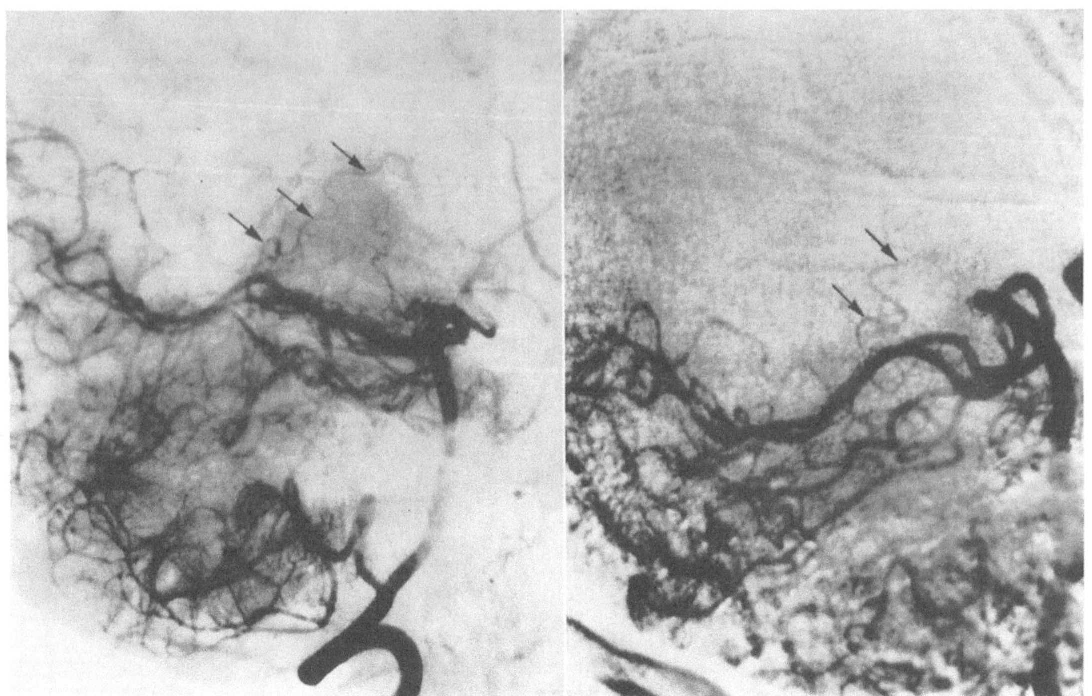

Fig. 21
Postero-medial dolicho-artery as well as cerebellar dolicho-arteries

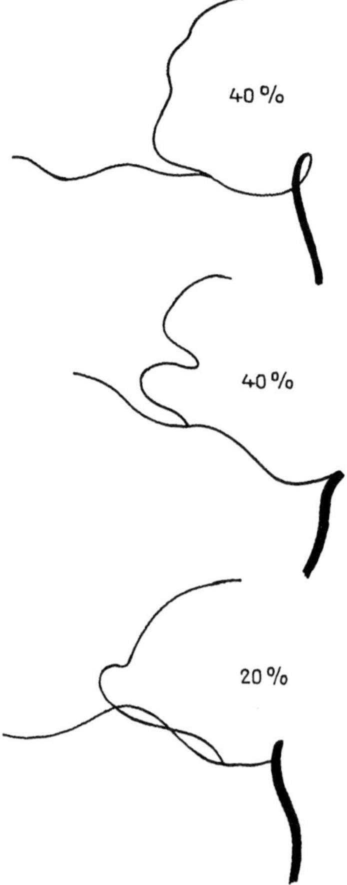

Fig. 22
Arteria chorioidea postero-medialis

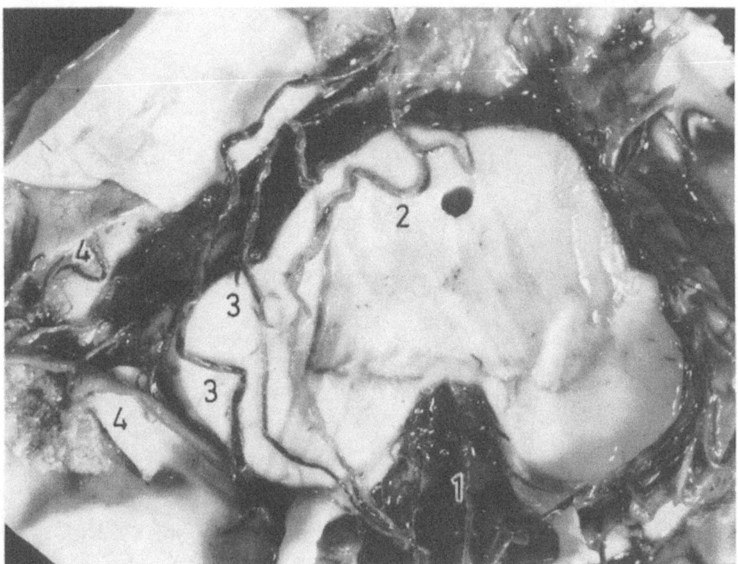

Fig. 23. Dissection of the mesencephalic arteries. *1* Posterior thalamo-perforating arteries. *2* Postero-medial choroidal artery. *3* Colliculi quadrigemini et corpori geniculati arteries. *4* Postero-lateral choroidal artery

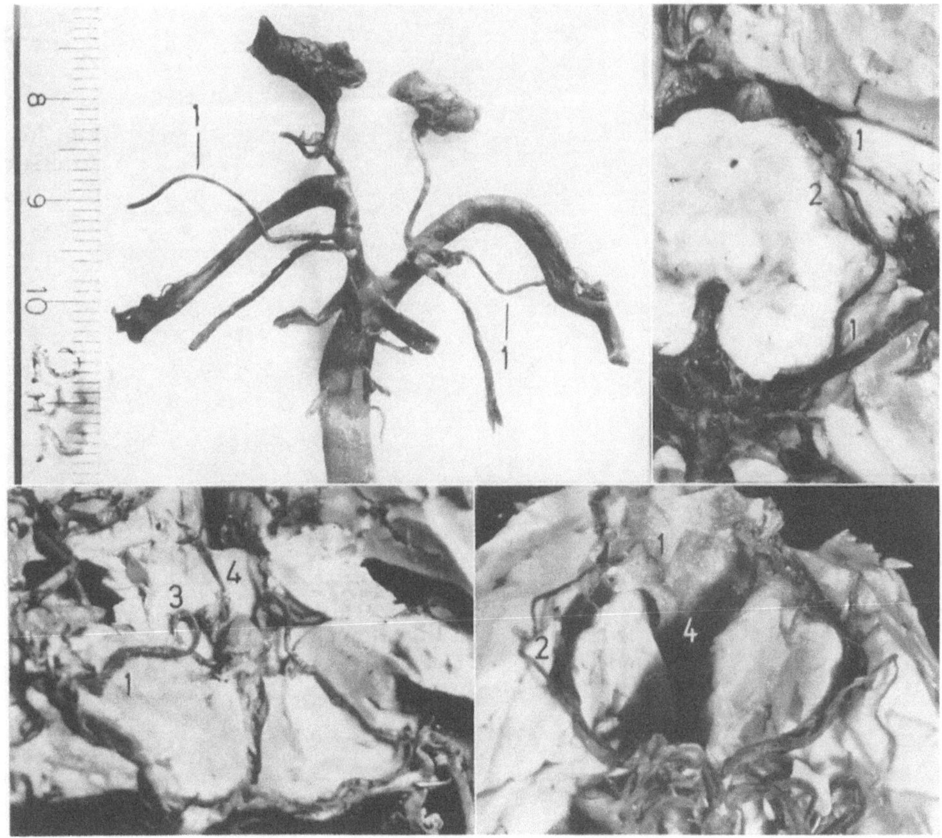

Fig. 24. The postero-medial choroidal artery (*1*) describes a loop at the level of the mesencephalic fissure (*2*) and yet another in the latero-pineal region (*3*) before coursing towards the choroidal plexus of the IIIrd ventricle (*4*)

63

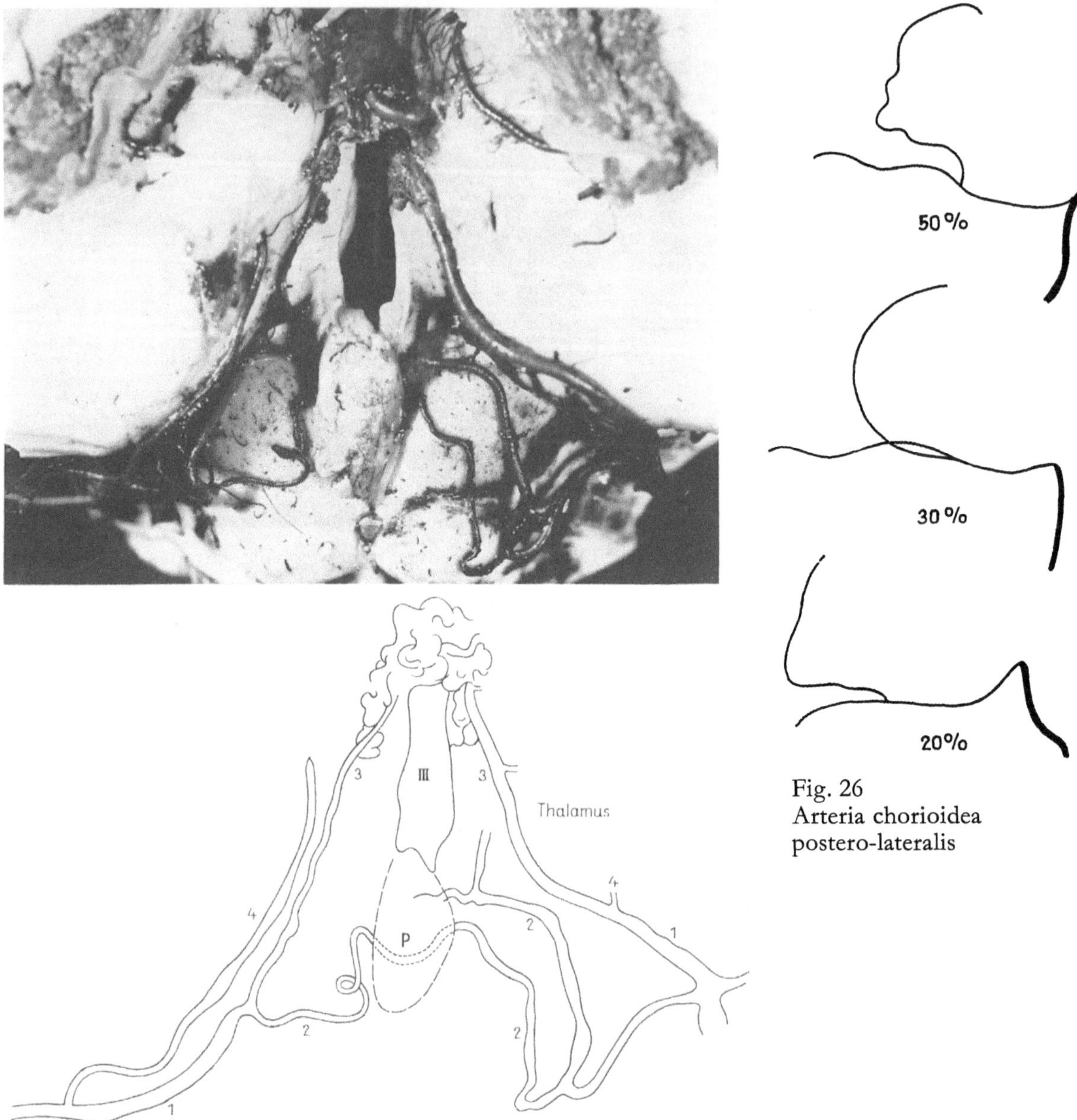

Fig. 26
Arteria chorioidea
postero-lateralis

Fig. 25
Dissection of the postero-medial choroidal artery: *1* Postero-medial
choroidal artery. *2* Pineal branch of the postero-medial choroidal artery
which may be at the origin of the pathological hammock shape of pinealomas (see Fig. 81). *3* Choroidal branch. *4* Thalamic branch

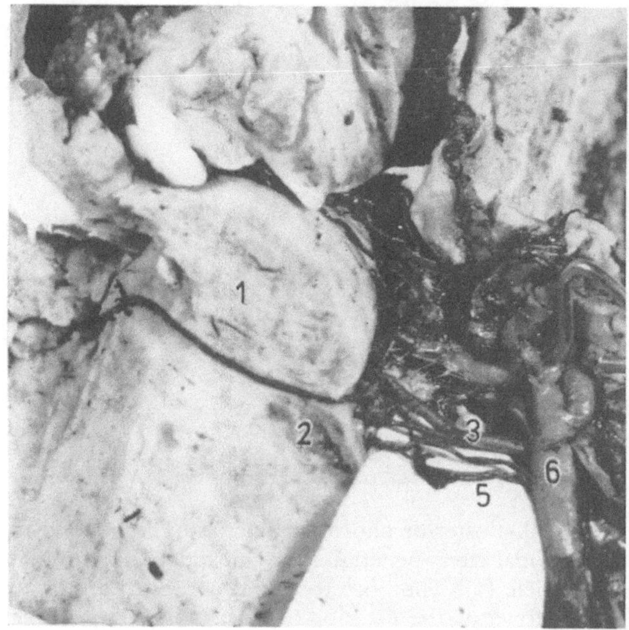

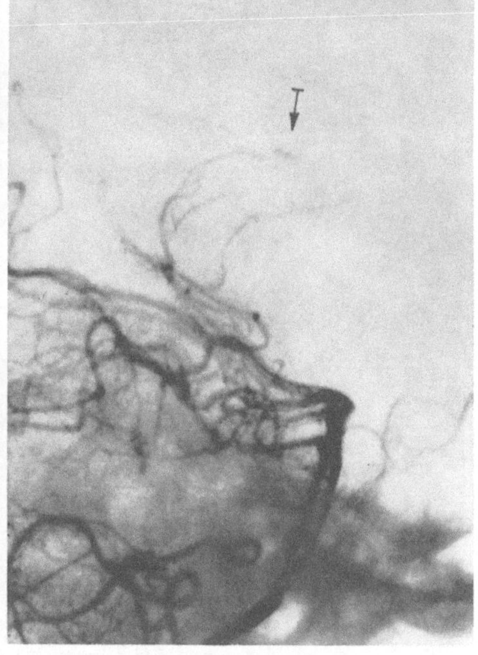

Fig. 28. On a lateral vertebral angiography several postero-lateral choroidal branches can be observed. Certain ones end in a cloud-like opacity corresponding to the choroidal plexus of the lateral ventricle

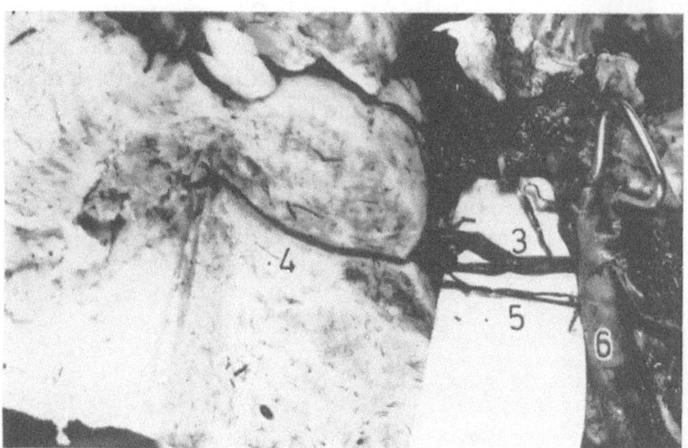

Fig. 27
Dissection of the postero-lateral choroidal artery:
1 Thalamus.
2 Lateral geniculate body.
3 Postero-lateral choroidal artery.
4 Thalamic branch of the postero-lateral choroidal artery.
5 Artery of the geniculate body.
6 Posterior cerebral artery

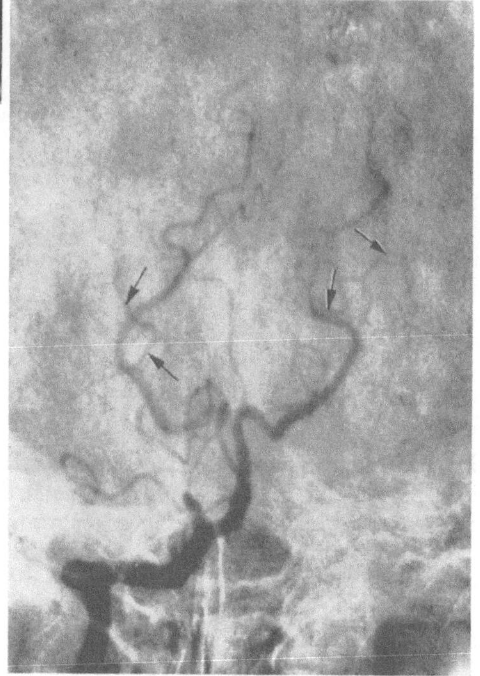

Fig. 29
Frontal projection of the postero-lateral choroidal artery

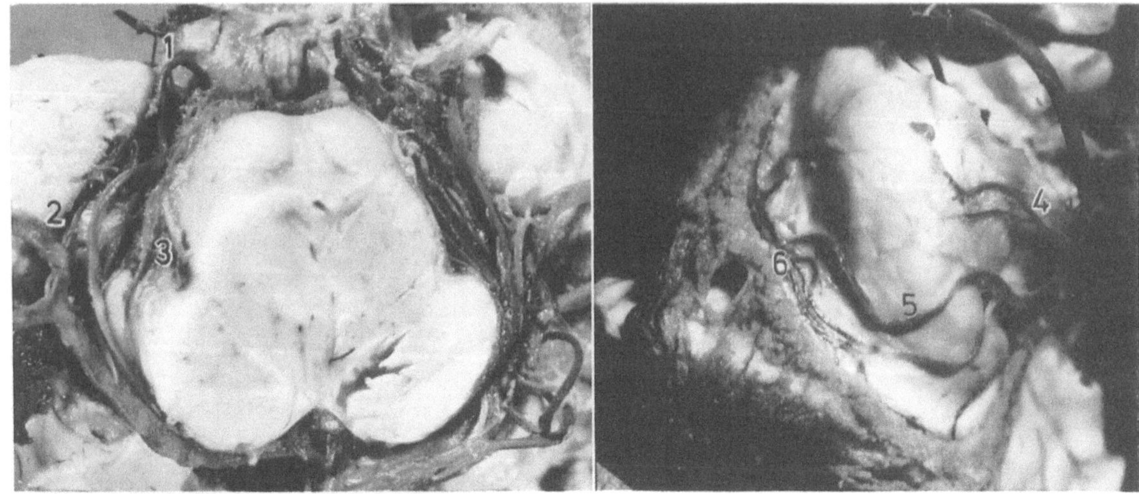

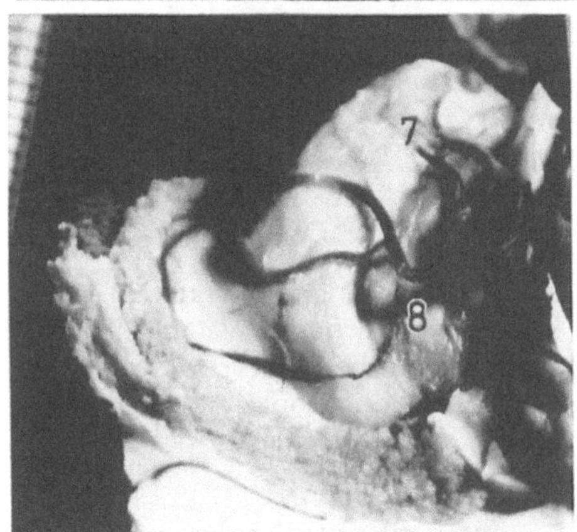

Fig. 30. Posterior choroidal arteries. The postero-medial choroidal artery penetrates the choroidal plexus of the IIIrd ventricle (*1*). The postero-lateral choroidal artery is situated towards the exterior (*2*). The colliculi quadrigemini artery describes a figure "3" whose midpoint corresponds to the mesencephalic fissure (*3*). The postero-lateral choroidal artery forks into a superior branch which penetrates the posterior thalamus (*4*) and an inferior branch which joins the choroidal plexus of the lateral ventricle (*5*). Generally it is this branch that we recognize on an angiogram. In this particular case it divides into four terminal branches (*6*). Superior postero-lateral choroidal artery (*7*), inferior postero-lateral choroidal artery divided in three terminal branches (*8*)

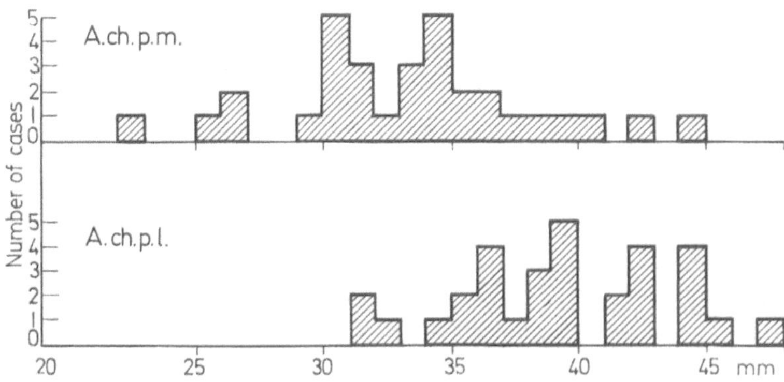

Fig. 31
Diagram of the statistical distribution of the distance separating the extremity of the basilar trunk from the farthest point of the postero-medial choroidal artery (upper diagram) and the postero-lateral (lower diagram) in 100 normal angiograms. Variations are more considerable at the level of the postero-medial choroidal than at the level of the postero-lateral choroidal arteries. Average values go from 30 to 35 mm for the postero-medial choroidal artery and 40 mm for the postero-lateral choroidal artery

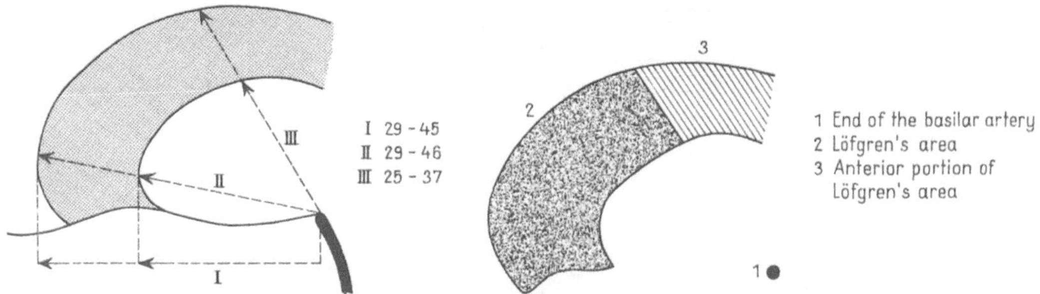

Fig. 32. Löfgren's diagram slightly modified (zone of lateral projection of the posterior choroidal arteries). This diagram is superimposed on the angiogram in some of our figures

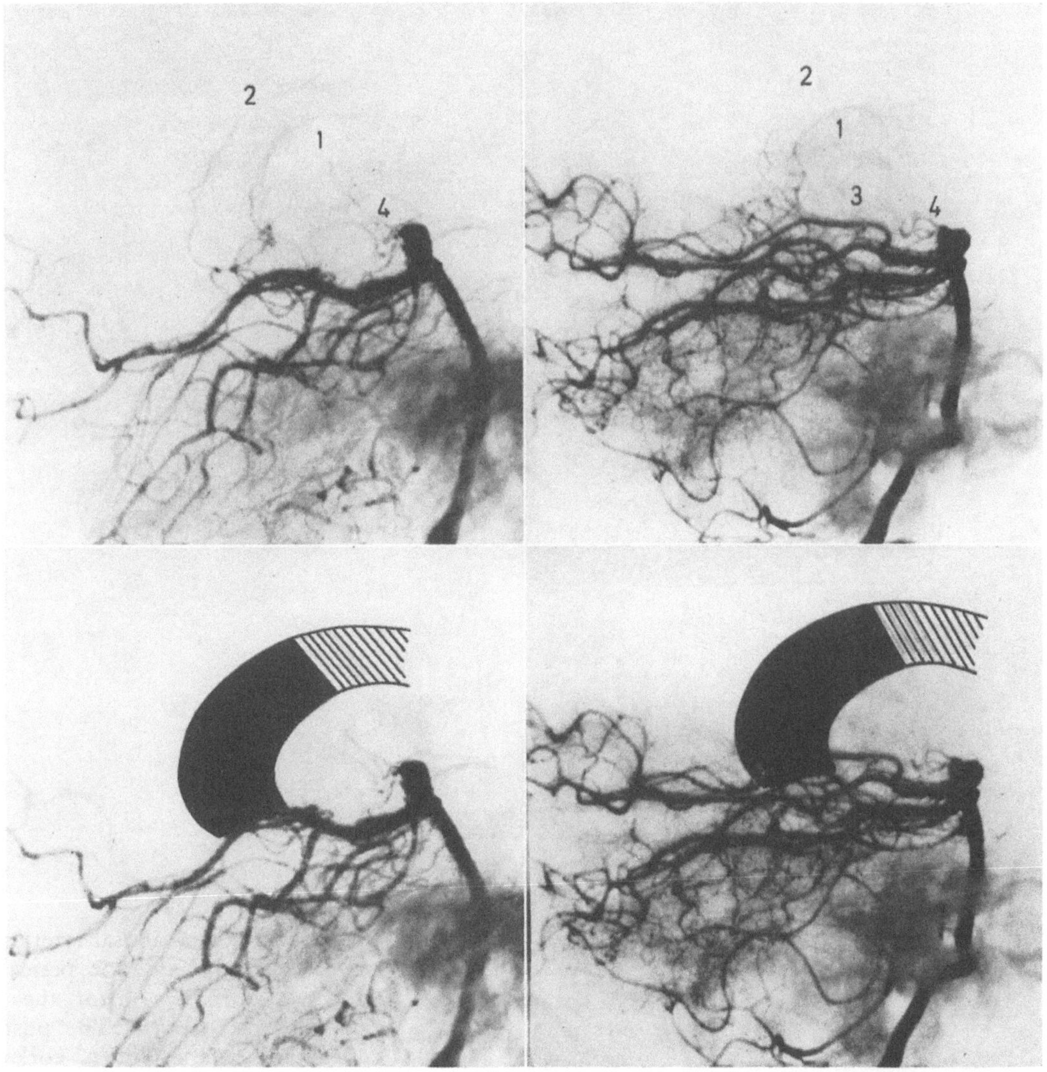

Fig. 33. Position of the arteries with relation to the diagram in two normal cases. Top: *1* Postero-medial choroidal artery. *2* Postero-lateral choroidal artery. *3* Colliculi quadrigemini and corpori geniculati arteries. *4* Posterior thalamo-perforating arteries. Bottom: The superimposition of the arterial diagram on the angiogram shows that the arteries are entirely covered

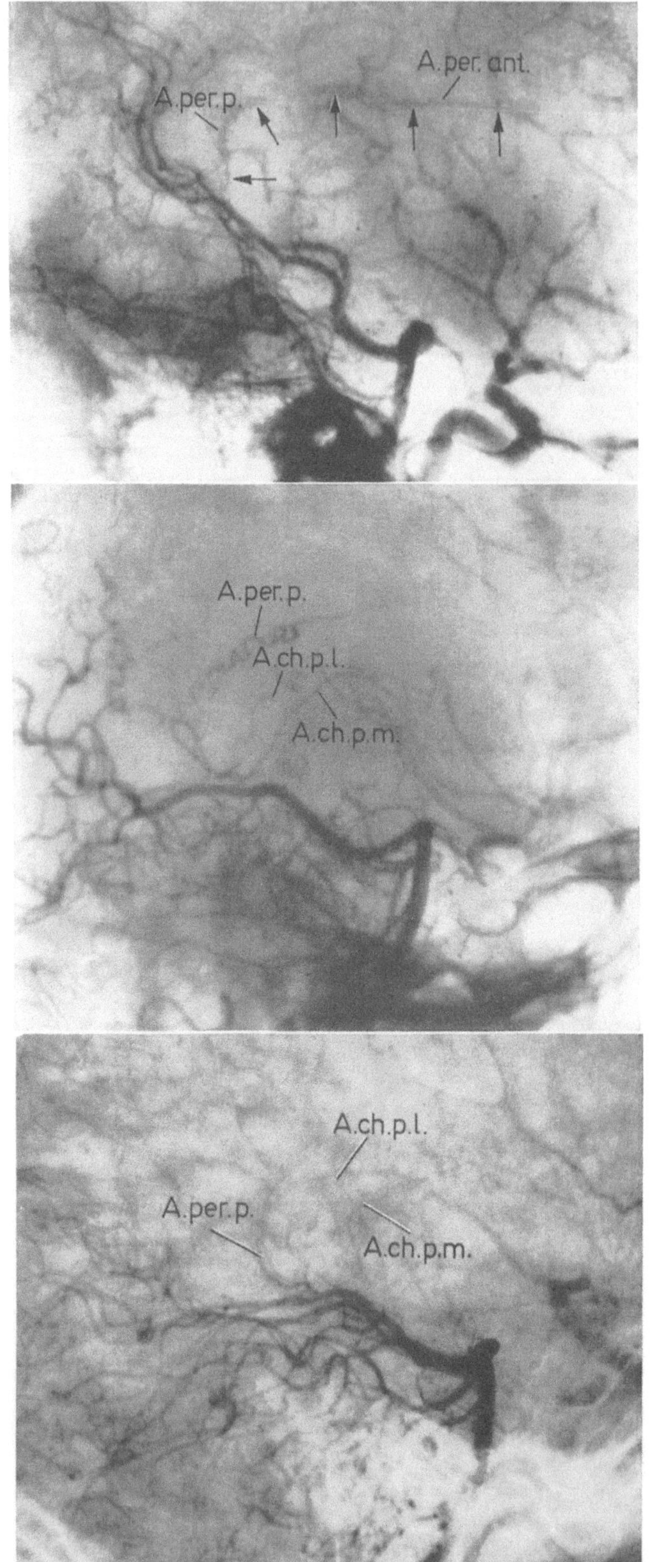

Fig. 34
The posterior pericallosal arteries (together with the anterior pericallosal artery). *Top:* They form the pericallosal circle. *Center:* The posterior pericallosal arteries in a corkscrew shape. This form is rare but normal. *Bottom:* The right and left posterior pericallosal arteries

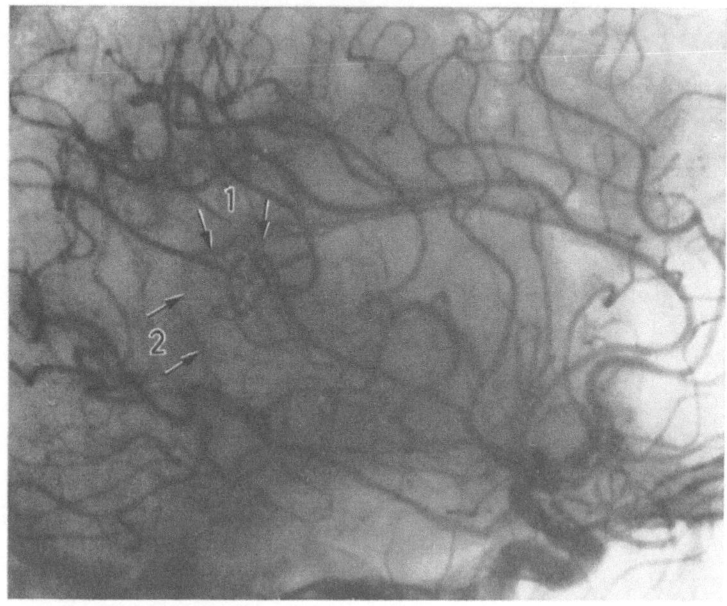

Fig. 35
Carotid angiography with opacification of the anterior pericallosal artery (*1*) and the posterior pericallosal artery (*2*)

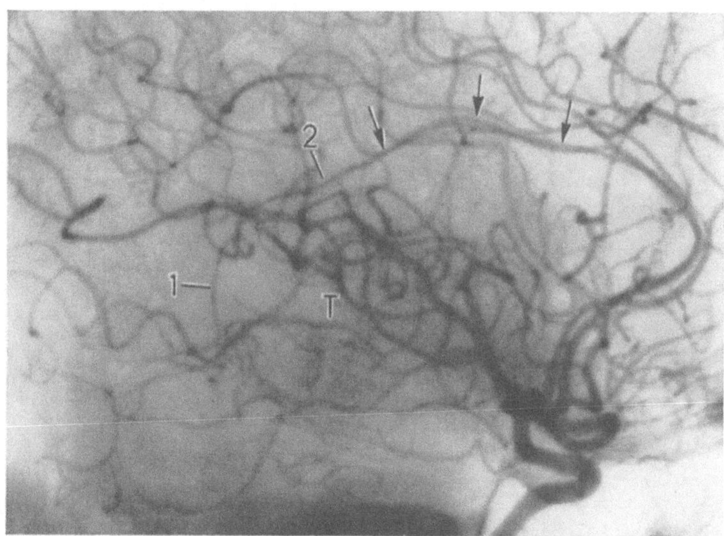

Fig. 36
A false pericallosal circle caused by a thalamo-peduncular tumour (*T*). The artery which *prolongs* the anterior pericallosal artery (*2*) is not the posterior pericallosal artery but the postero-lateral choroidal artery (*1*) displaced backward by the tumour

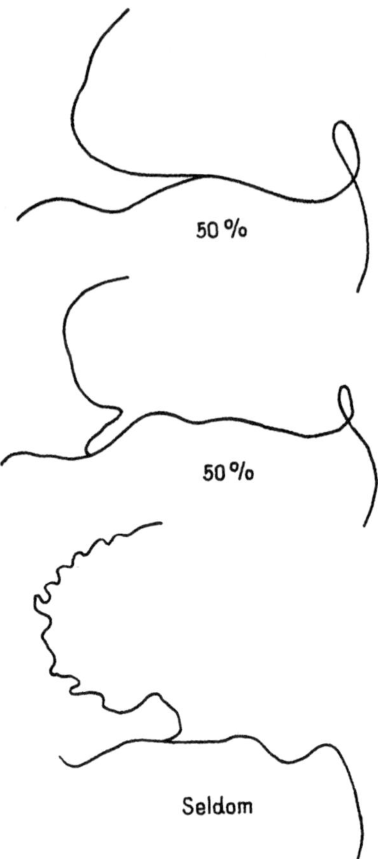

Fig. 37
Arteria pericallosa posterior

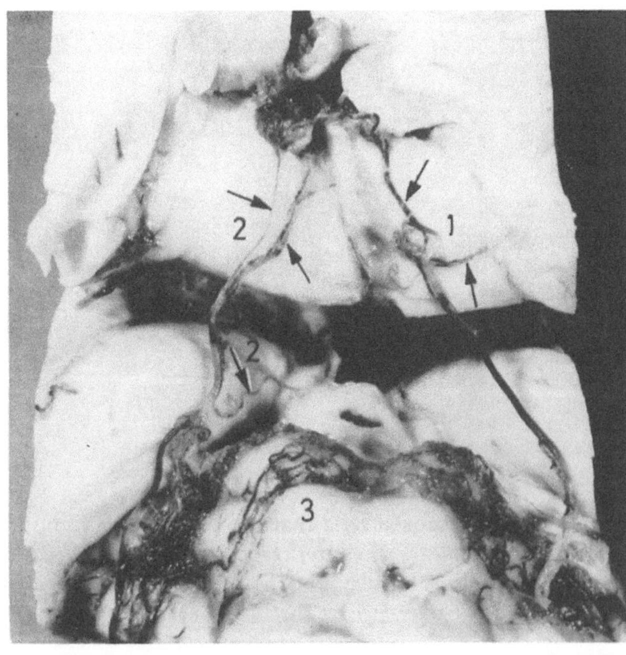

Fig. 38
The posterior pericallosal arteries follow a curvilineal course towards the splenium. In this case it divides into two terminal branches (*1*) on one side. The division in three branches on the other side is earlier (*2*); quadrigeminal bodies (*3*)

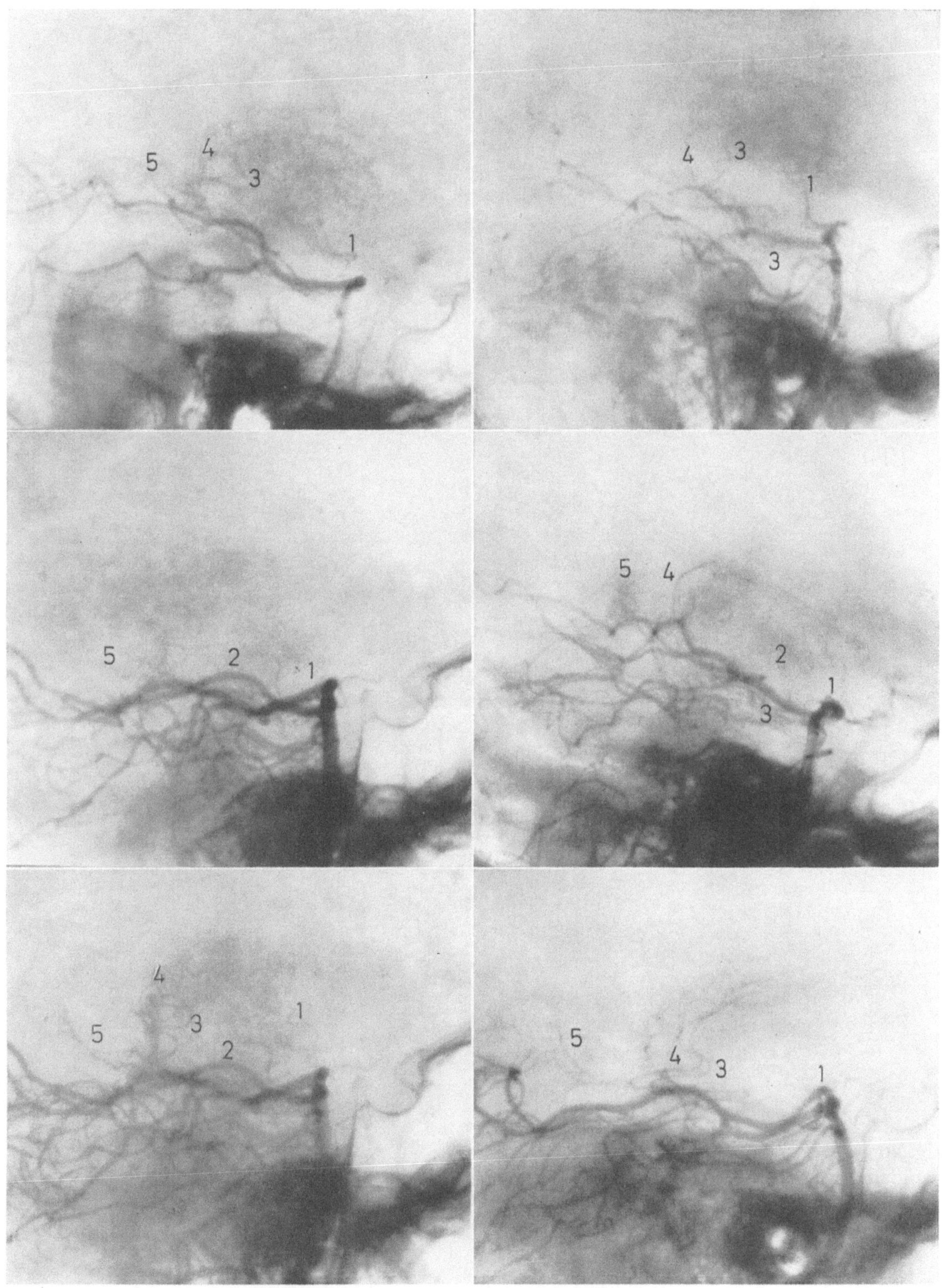

Fig. 39
Different types of mesencephalic arteries in lateral projection: *1* Posterior thalamo-perforating arteries. *2* Colliculi-quadrigemini arteries. *3* Postero-medial choroidal arteries. *4* Postero-lateral choroidal arteries. *5* Posterior pericallosal artery

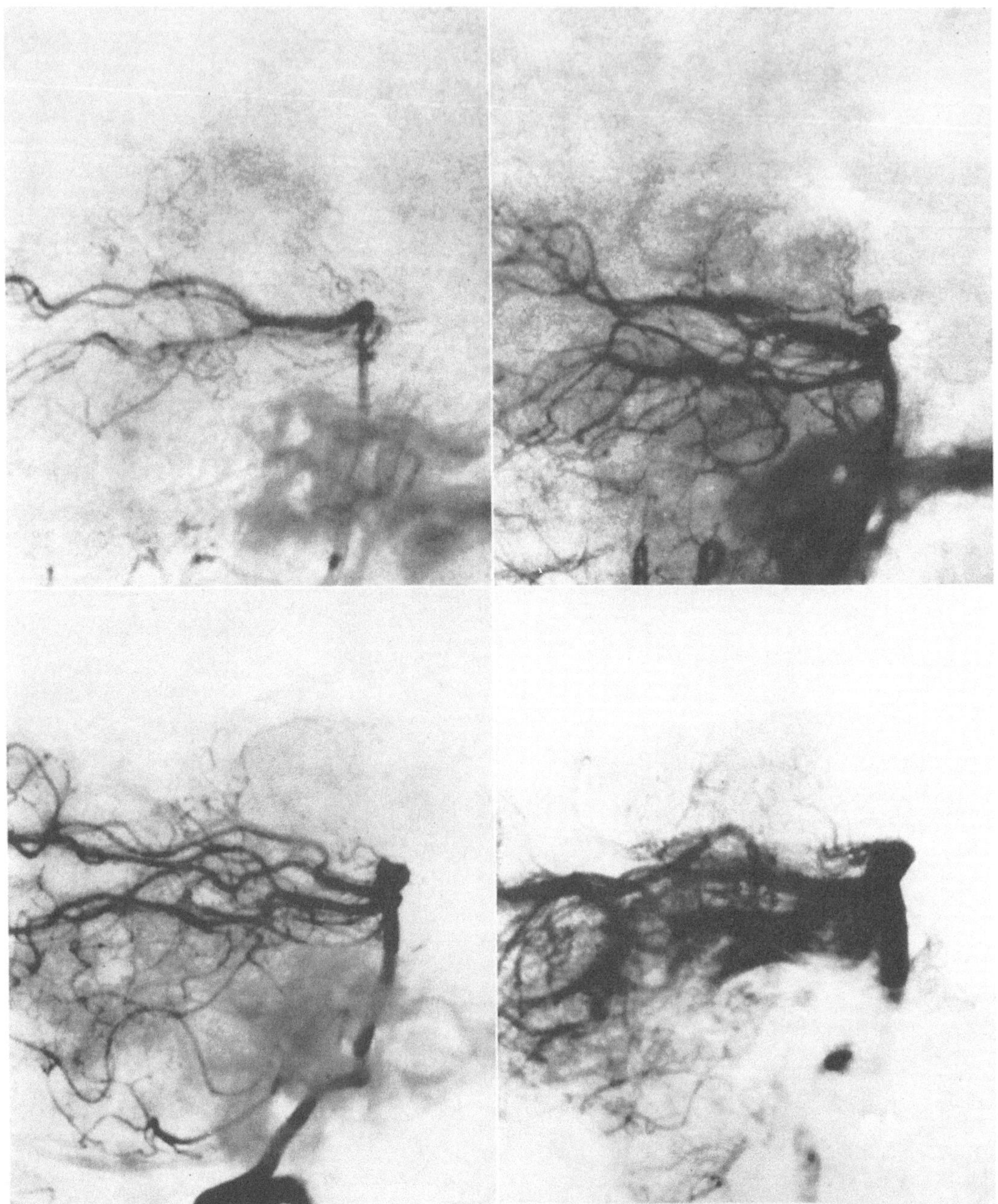

Fig. 40
Capillarography in the area of the mesencephalic arteries in lateral projection after subtraction

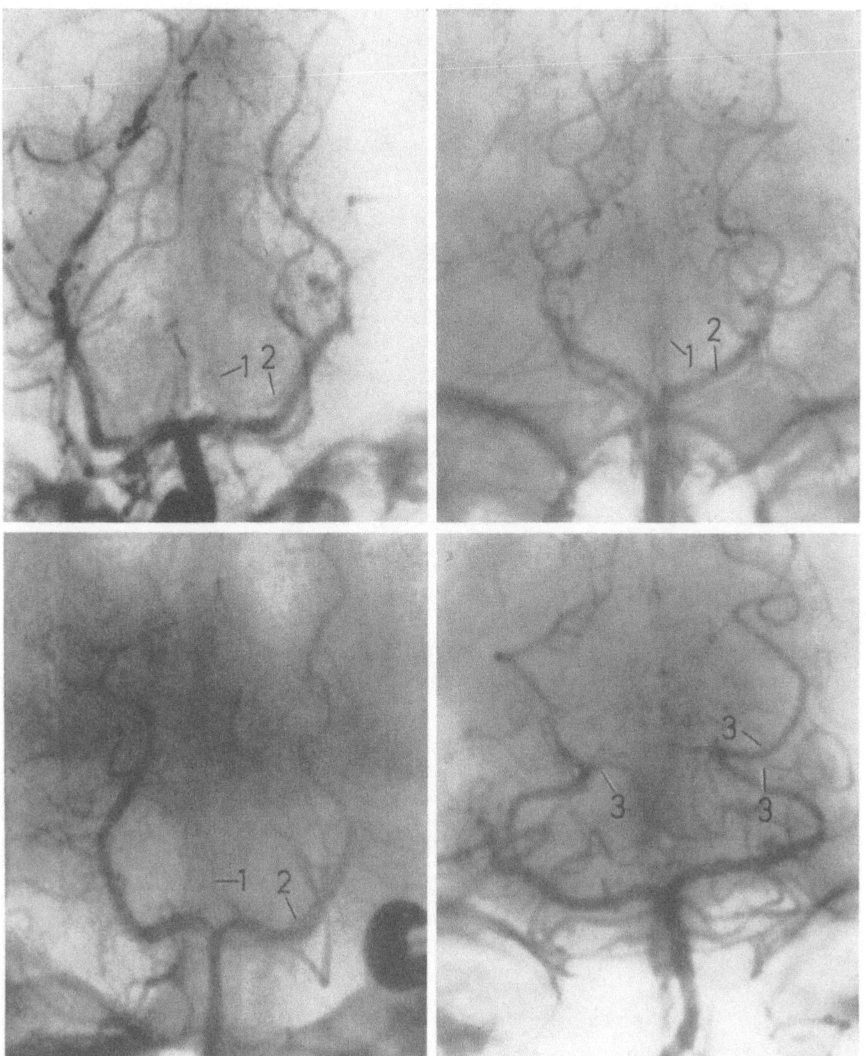

Fig. 41
Views of mesencephalic arteries in frontal projection on a conventional angiogram: *1* Thalamo-perforating arteries. *2* Postero-medial choroidal artery. *3* Postero-lateral choroidal artery

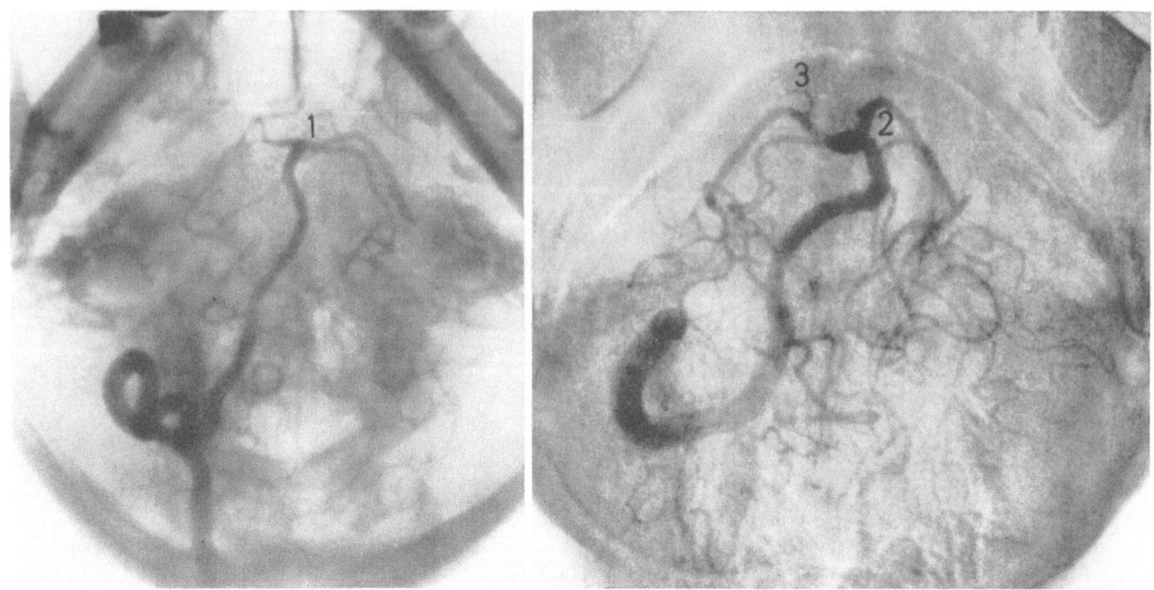

Fig. 42
Mesencephalic arteries are not easily identifiable in an axial view even in subtraction. *1* Posterior thalamo-perforating artery. *2* Postero-medial choroidal artery. *3* Posterior communicating artery

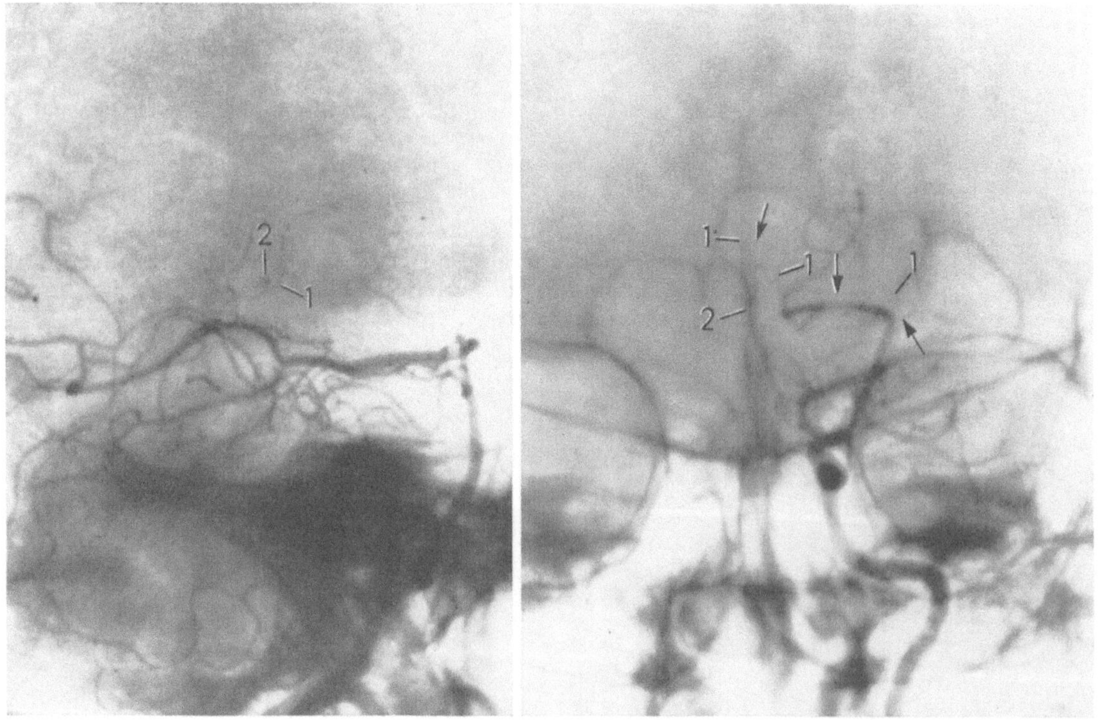

Fig. 43

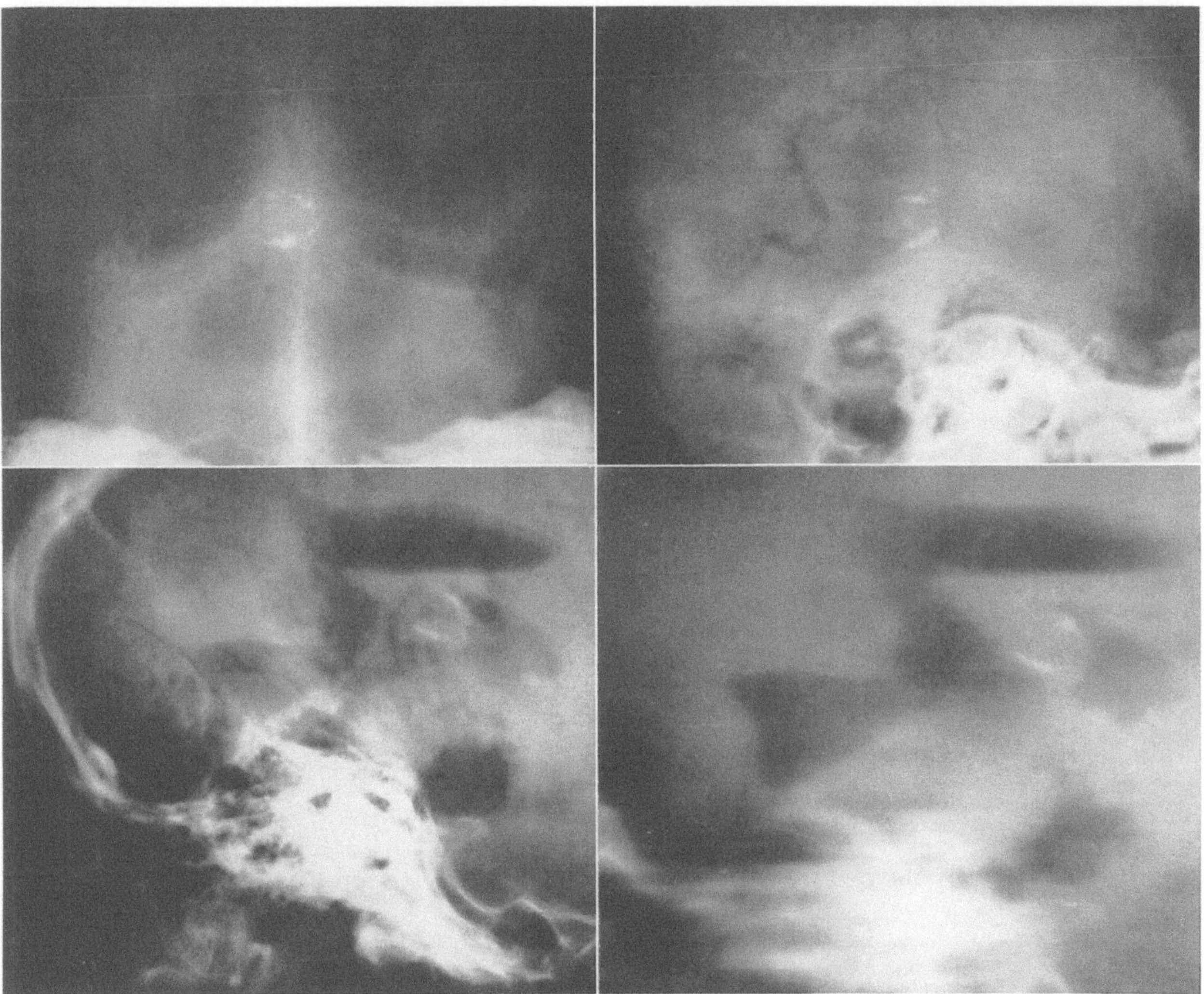

Fig. 44
Calcification surrounding a small pinealoma. *Top :* Plain radiogram. *Bottom :* Pneumo-encephalography on
the left and stratigraphy on the right

Fig. 43
Relation of the calcified pineal gland with the posterior medial choroidal arteries. *Lateral view :*
1 Zone of inversion of curvature of the postero-medial choroidal artery. *2* Calcified pineal gland.
Frontal view : 1 Postero-medial choroidal artery (↑). *2* Calcified pineal gland

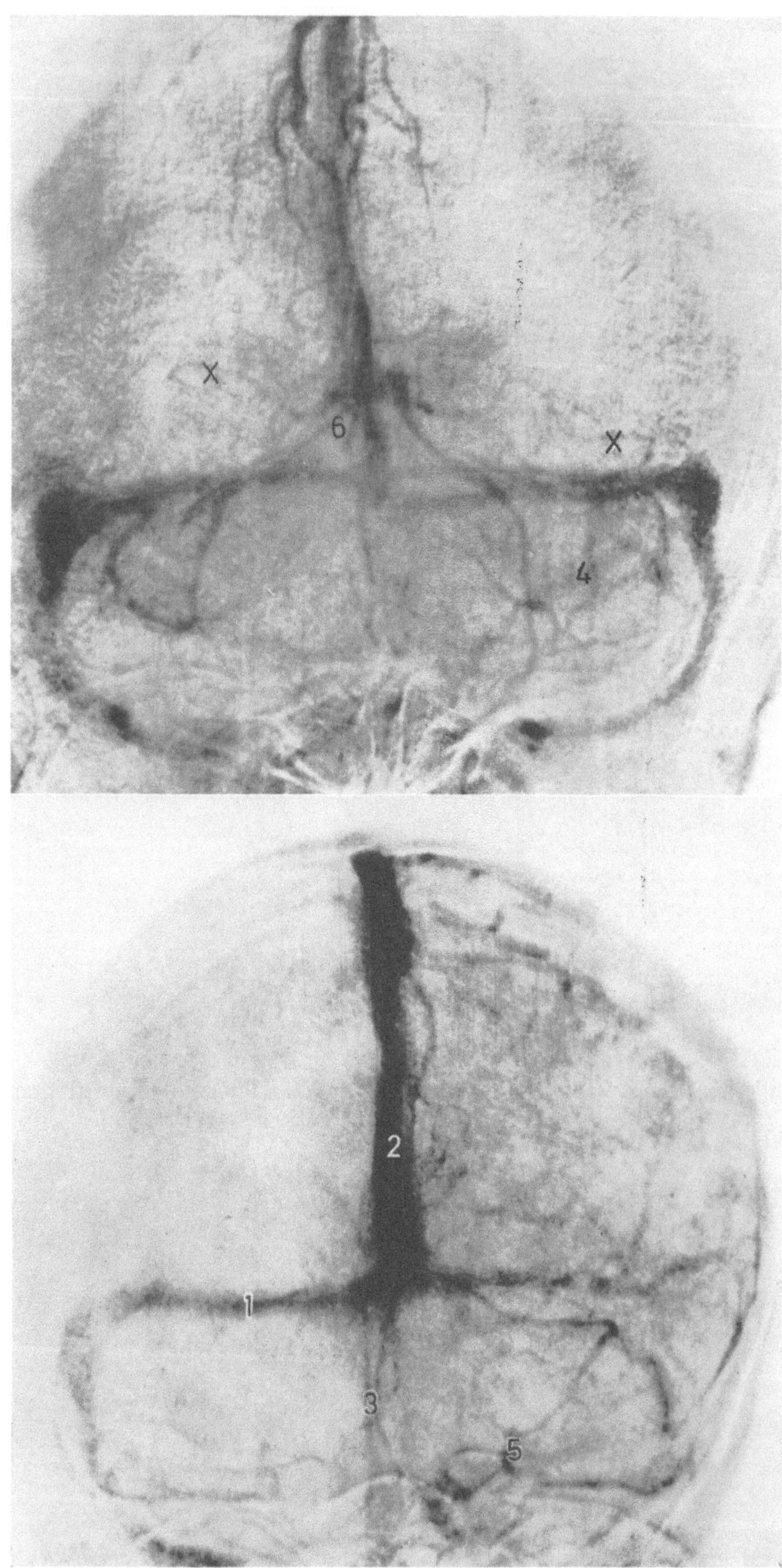

Fig. 45
Normal vertebral veno-
gram in frontal view.
1 Lateral sinus.
2 Longitudinal sinus.
3 Inferior vermian
  veins.
4 Hemispheric
  cerebellar veins.
5 Petrosal vein.
6 Precentral vein

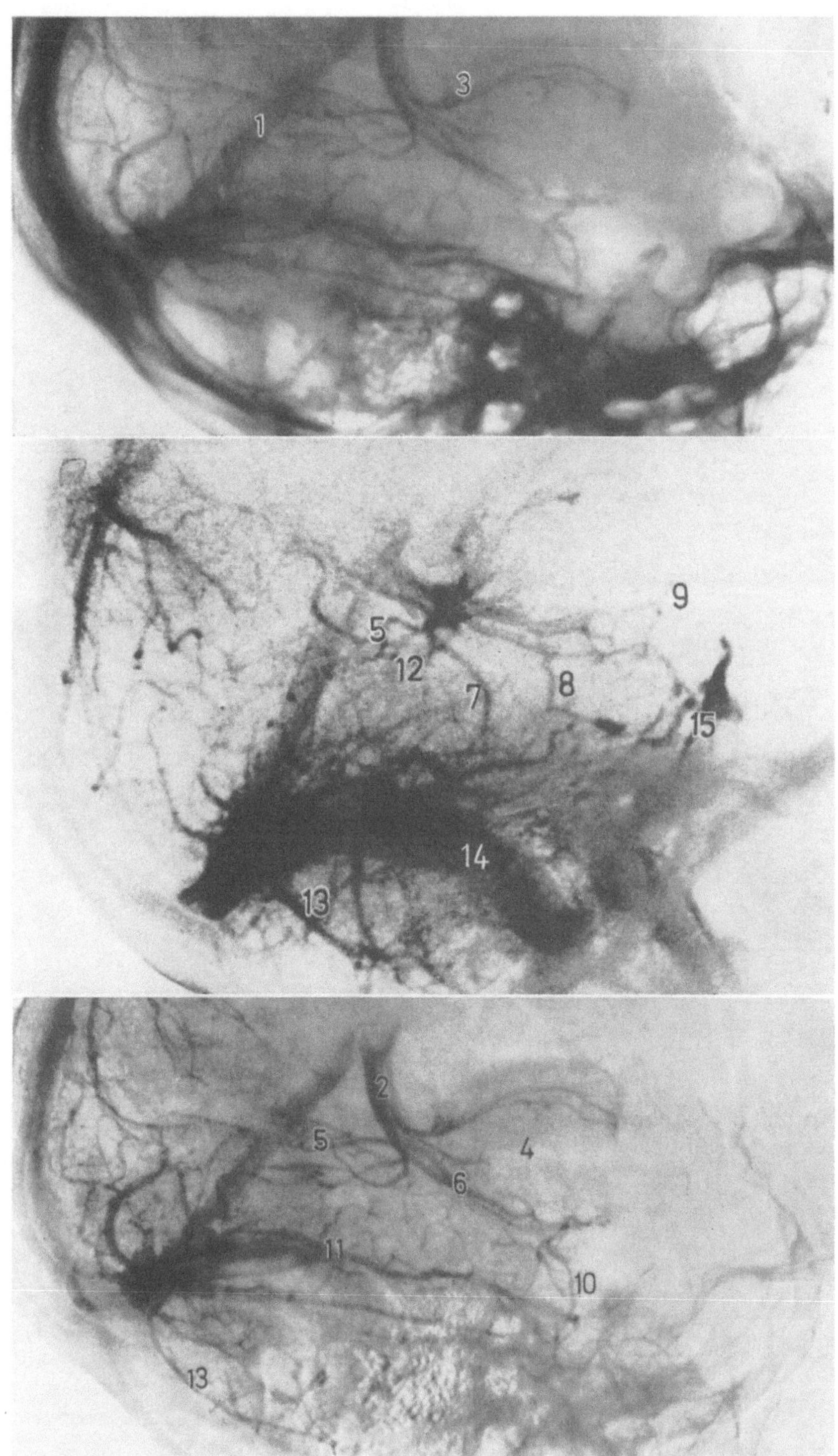

Fig. 46. Normal vertebral venogram in lateral view. *1* Straight sinus. *2* Great vein of Galen. *3* Internal cerebral vein. *4* Thalamic veins. *5* Occipital veins. *6* Basal vein. *7* Precentral vein. *8* Lateral mesencephalic vein. *9* Interpeduncular veins. *10* Prepontine veins. *11* Hemispheric cerebellar veins. *12* Superior vermian vein. *13* Inferior vermian vein. *14* Lateral sinus. *15* Clivus veins

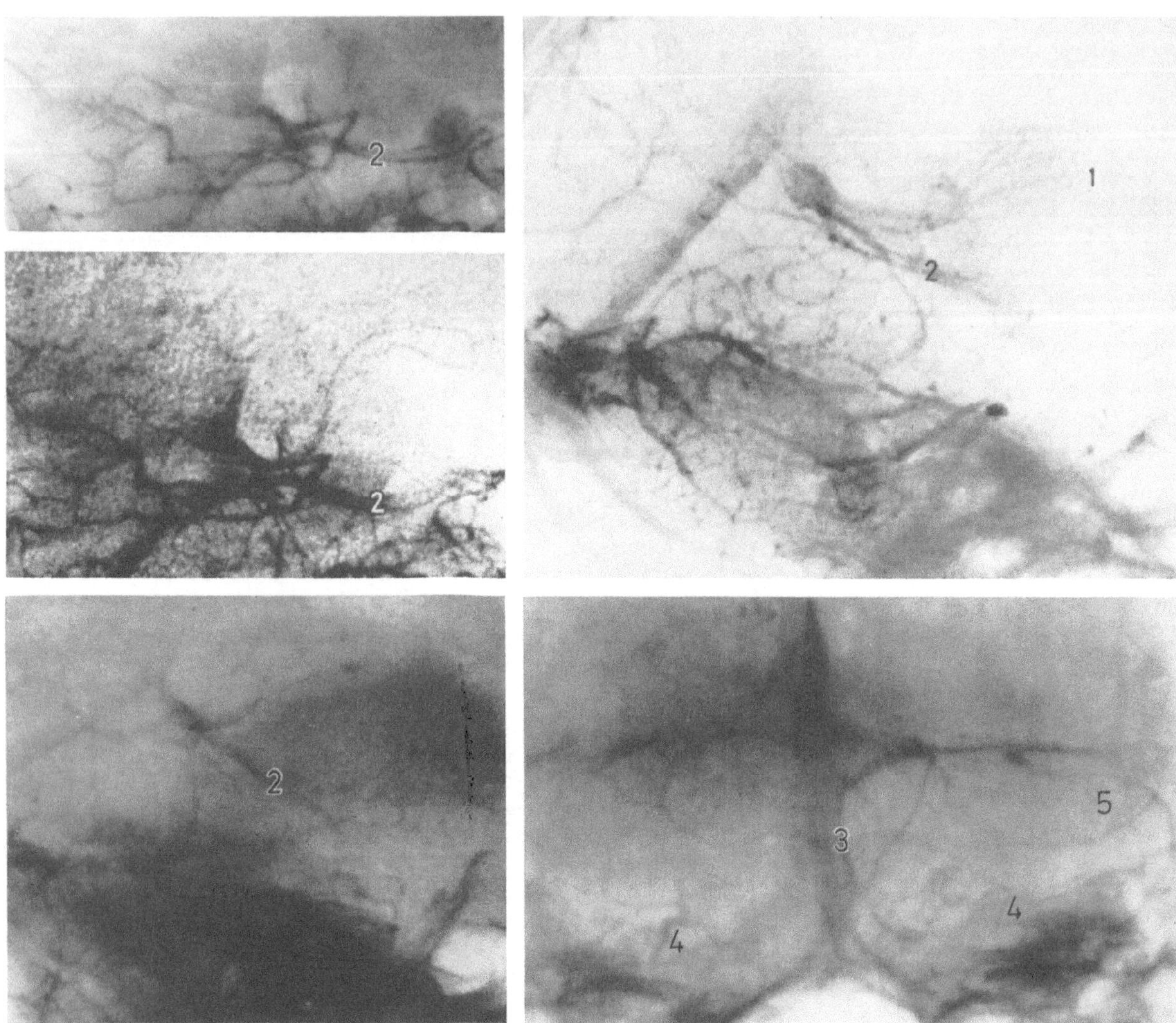

Fig. 47
Normal venogram. *1* Thalamic veins. *2* Posterior mesencephalic veins. *3* Inferior vermian vein. *4* Petrosal veins. *5* Hemispheric veins

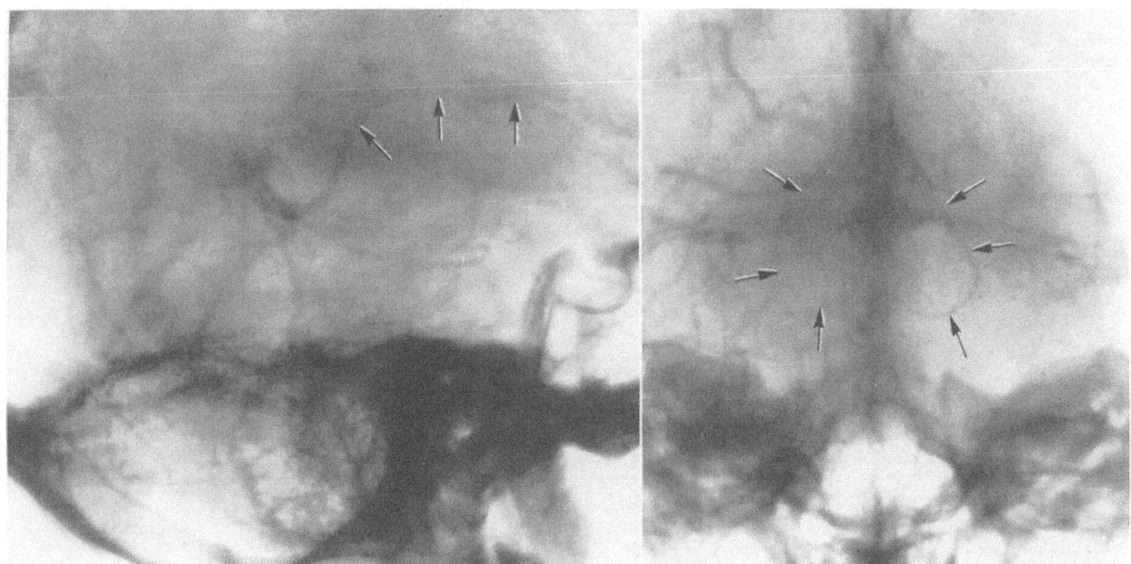

Fig. 48. Normal vertebral venogram. The internal cerebral vein is plainly opacified in this case (left). The brain stem is surrounded by the posterior mesencephalic veins (right)

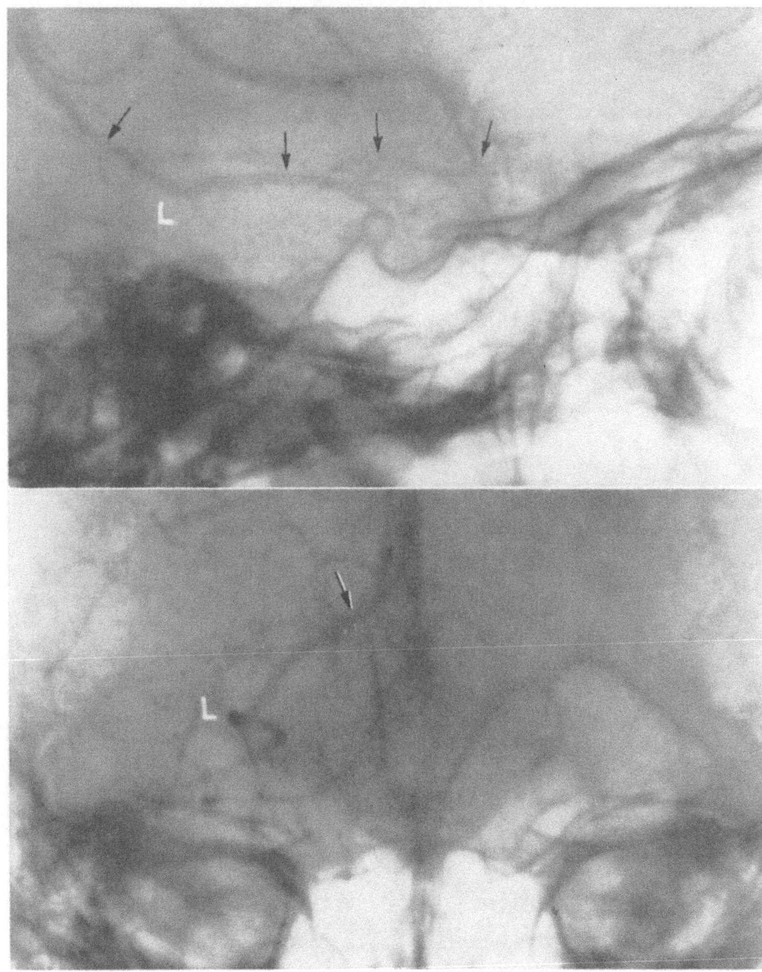

Fig. 49
We distinguished two parts of the basal vein: Anterior part courses parallel to the basal line of Virchow to point *L* which corresponds to the most external position of the vein near the brainstem. Posterior part joins the great vein of Galen in the ambient cistern

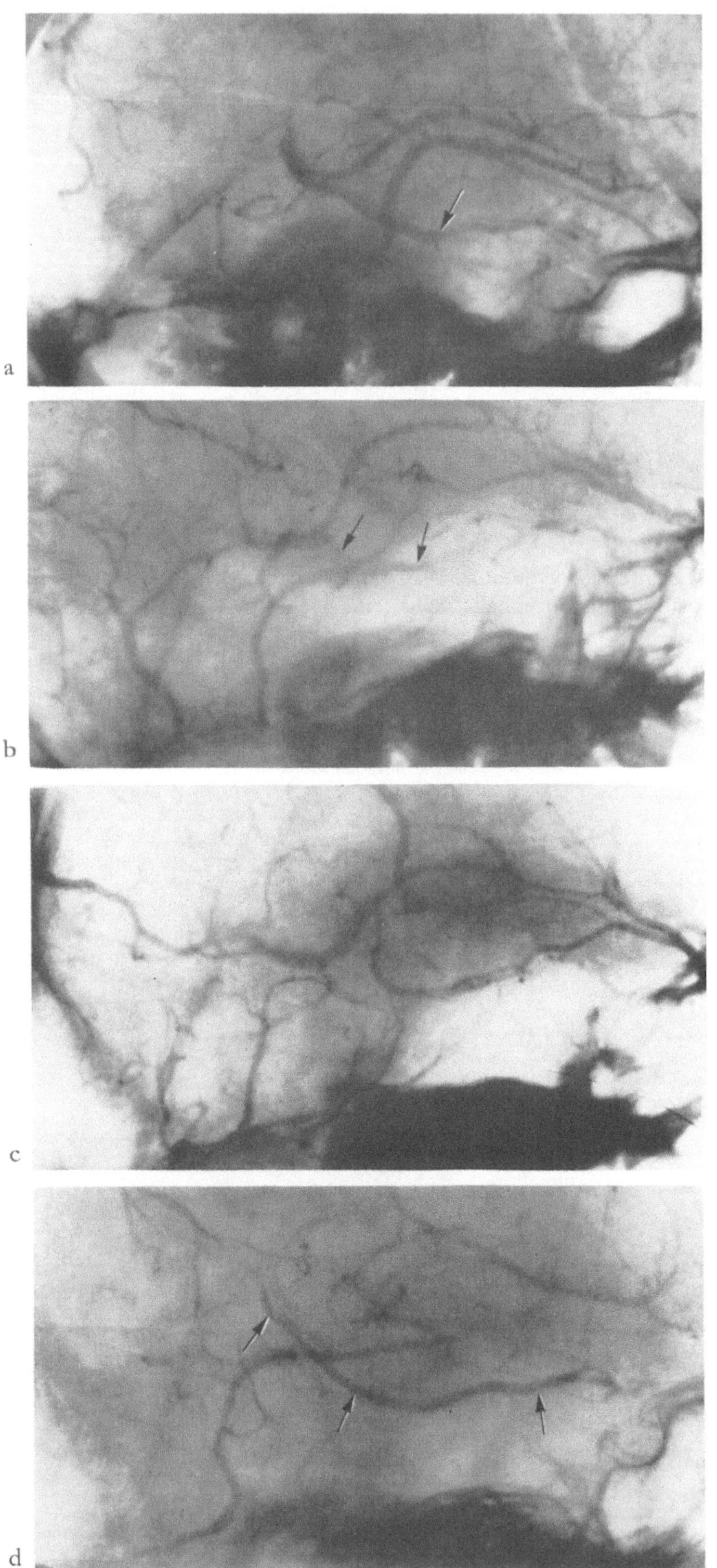

Fig. 50a–d
Variation of the basal vein.
a) Great variation in calibre at the level of point "L". b) The posterior segment alone of the basal vein is opacified. c) Absence of the basal vein. d) Dilatation of the basal vein which joins the right sinus

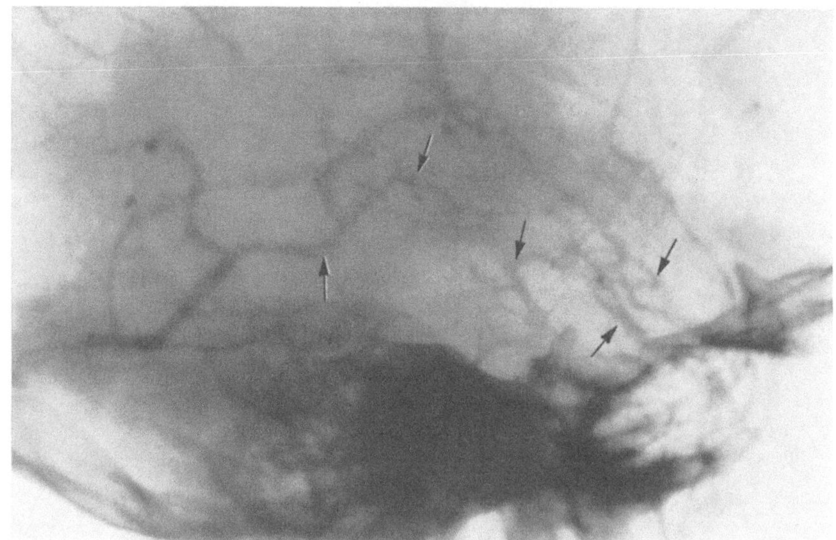

Fig. 51
Complex venous network which replaces the basal vein

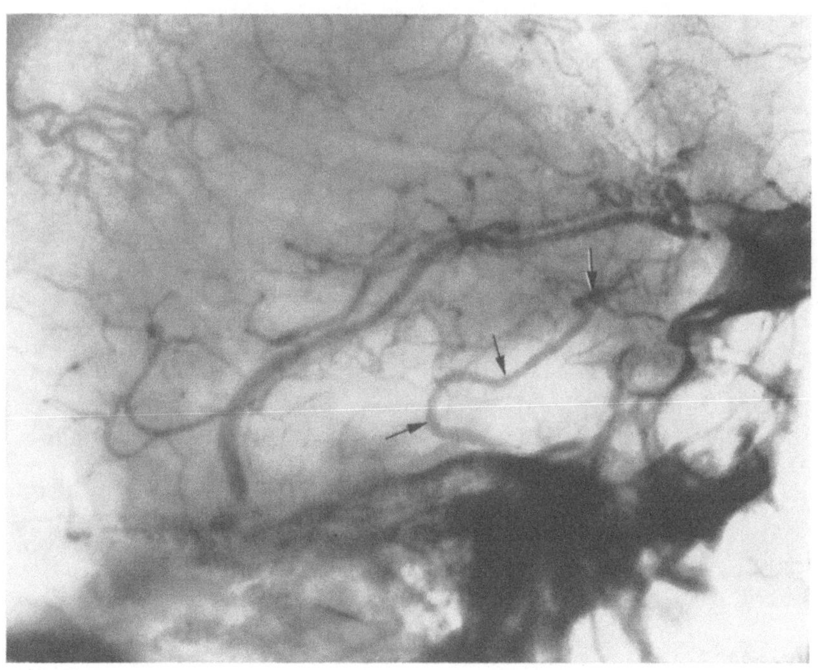

Fig. 52
Variation in venous drainage in the area of the basal vein

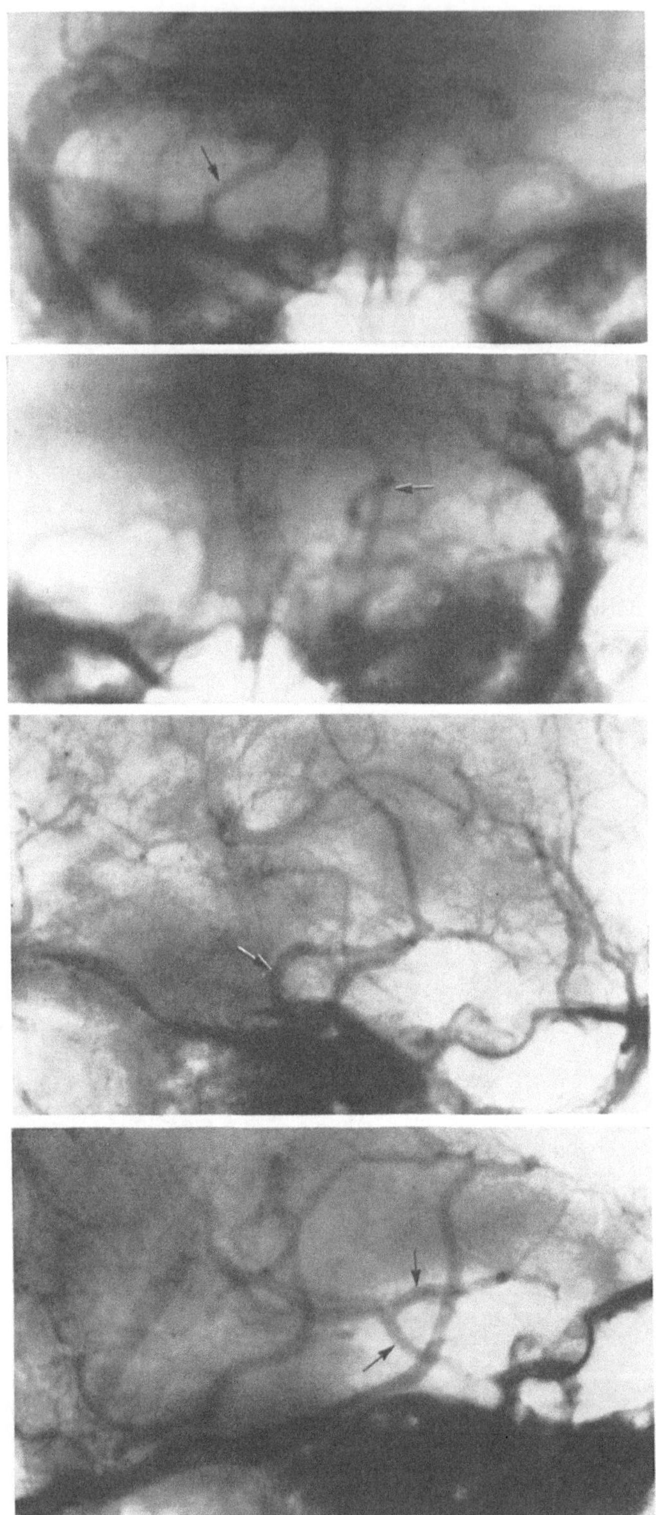

Fig. 53a

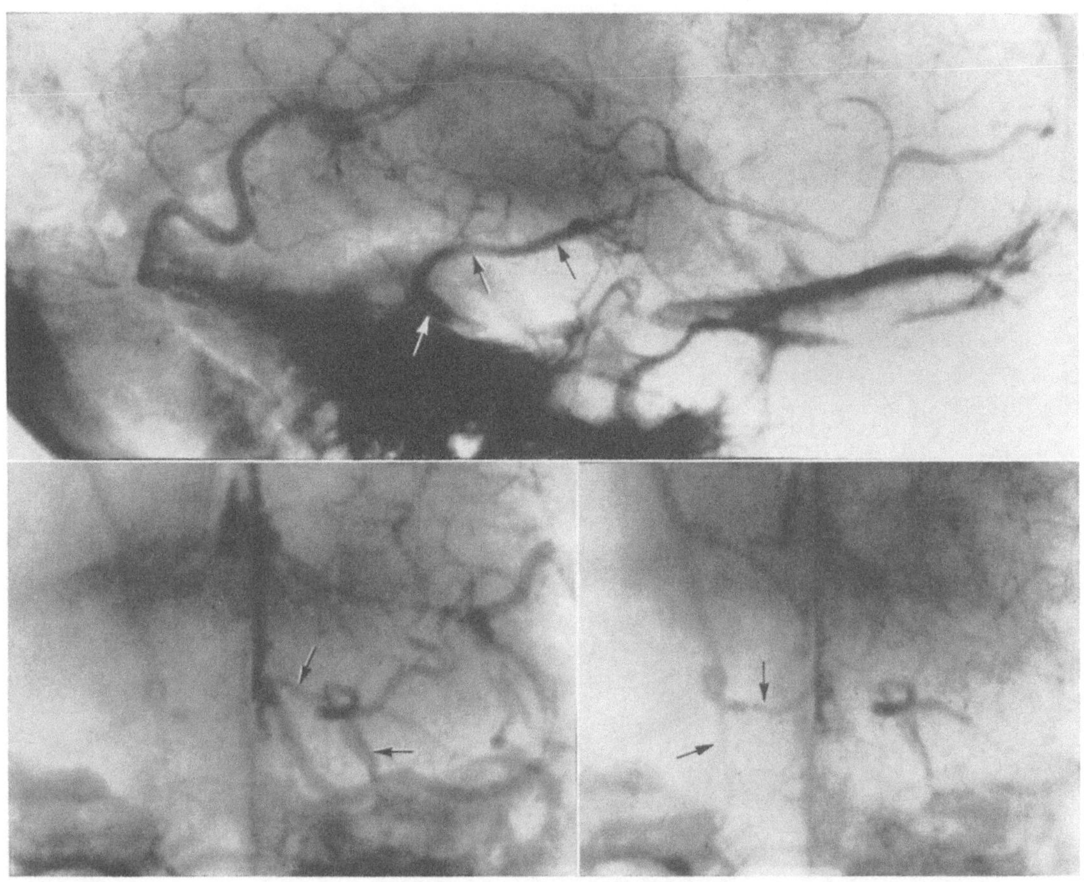

Fig. 53b

Fig. 53a and b
Two cases of a bilateral anastomotic mesencephalic vein

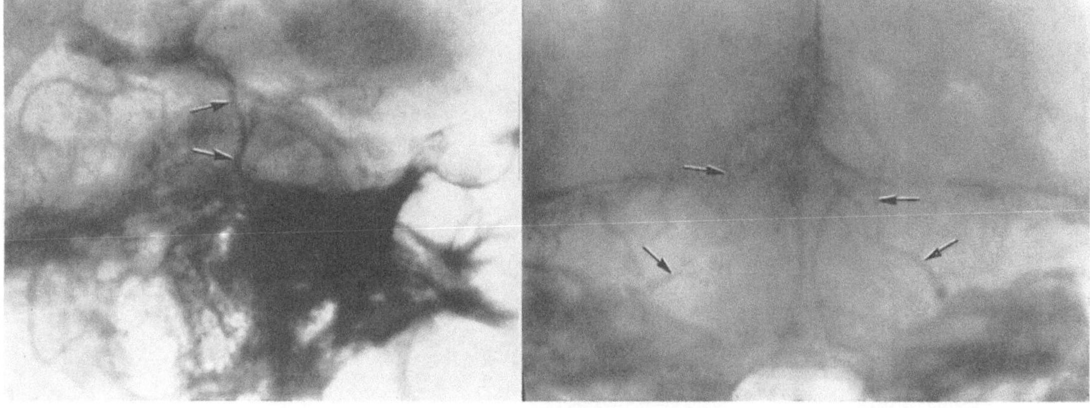

Fig. 54
An anterior bilateral cerebellar vein which outlines the brainstem

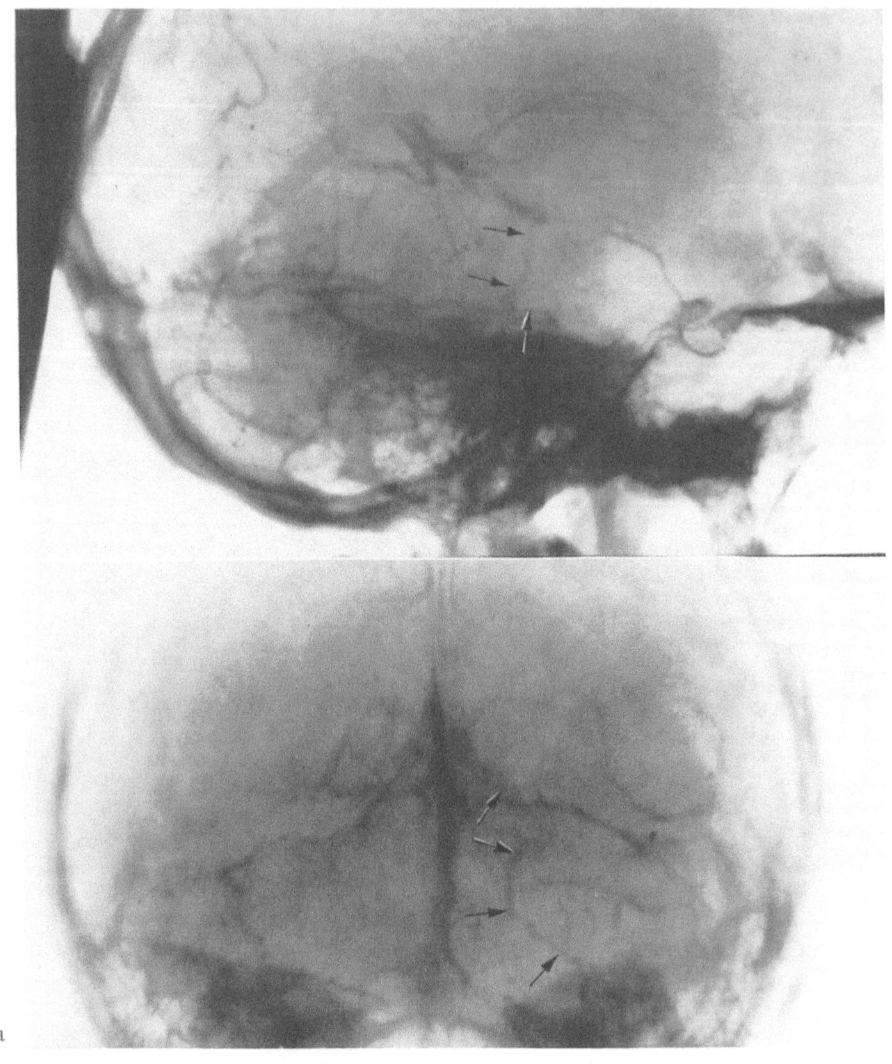

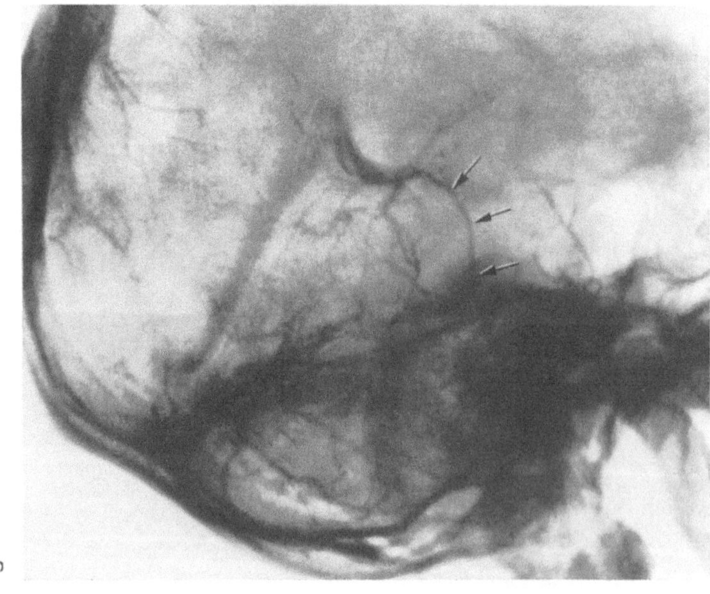

Fig. 55a and b
Two cases of the anterior cerebellar vein

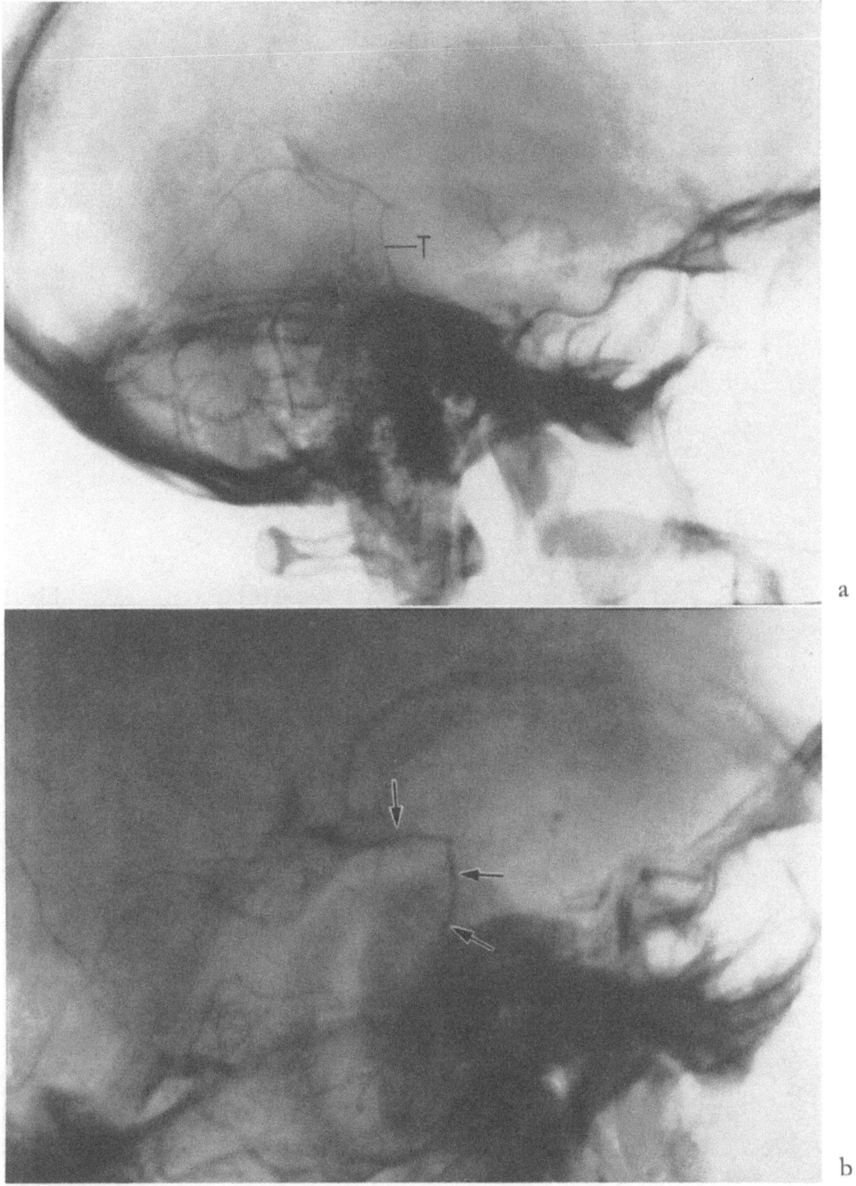

Fig. 56a and b
a) Craniopharyngioma which displaces the mesencephalic vein backwards
(anterior concavity of the vein). b) Normal anterior cerebellar vein. The
lateral mesencephalic segment is convex frontwards

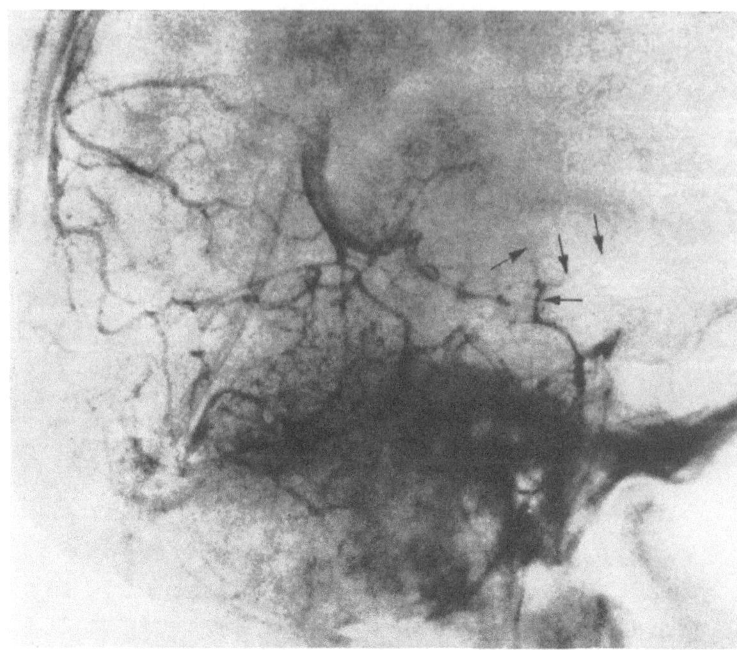

Fig. 57
Interpeduncular vein

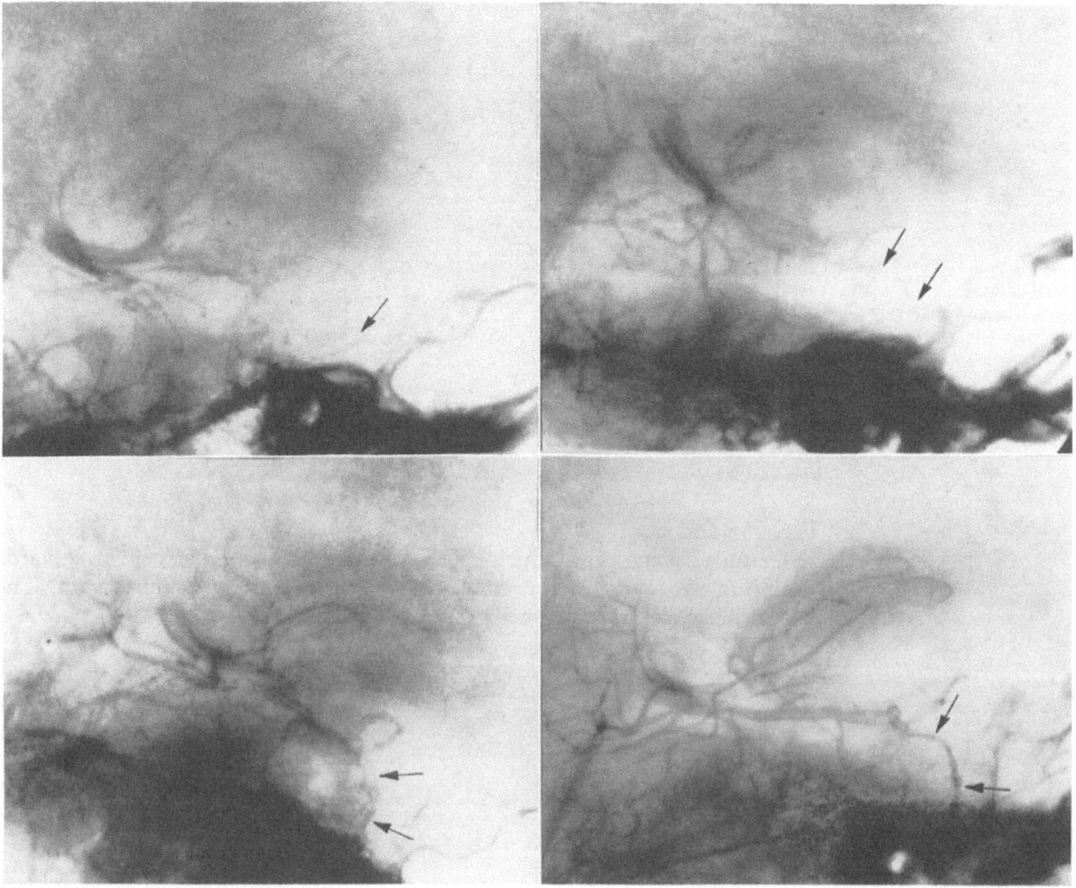

Fig. 58. Ponto-mesencephalic vein

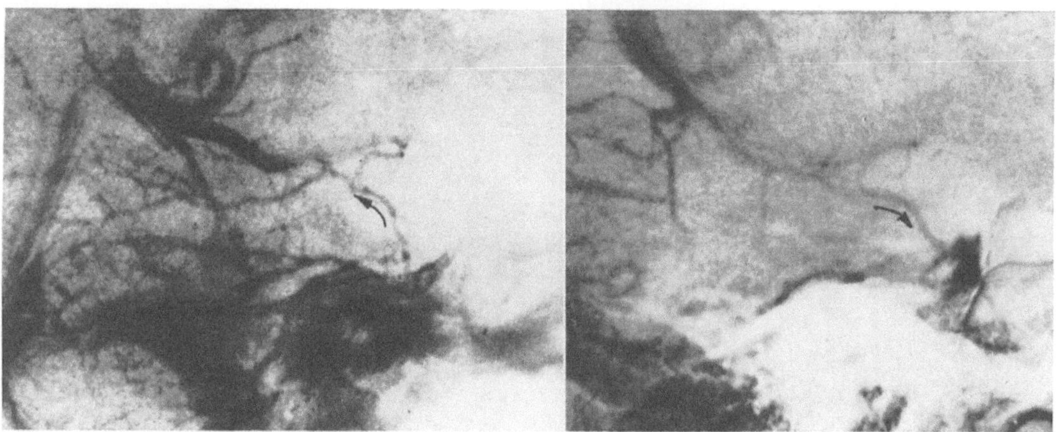

Fig. 59
Anterior and posterior drainage of the ponto-mesencephalic vein

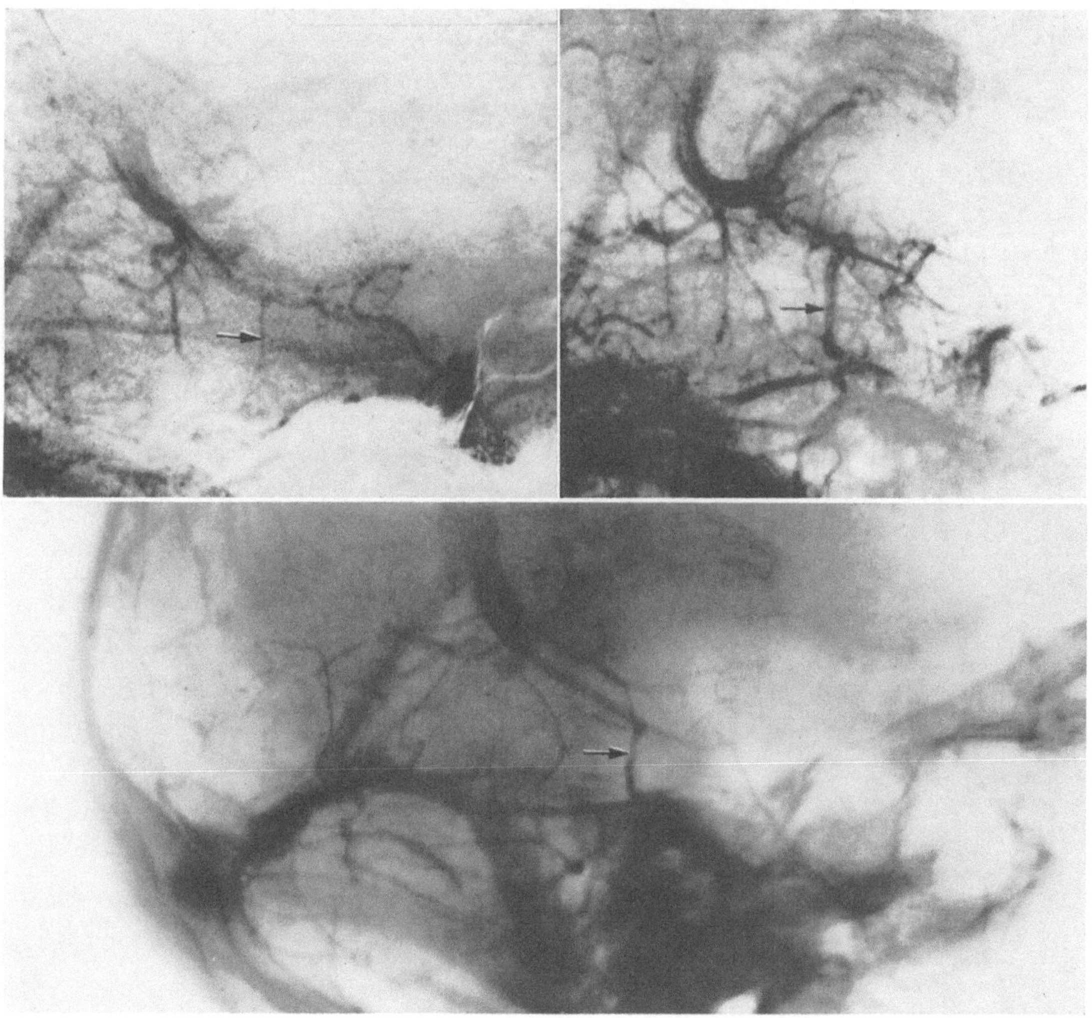

Fig. 60
Lateral mesencephalic vein

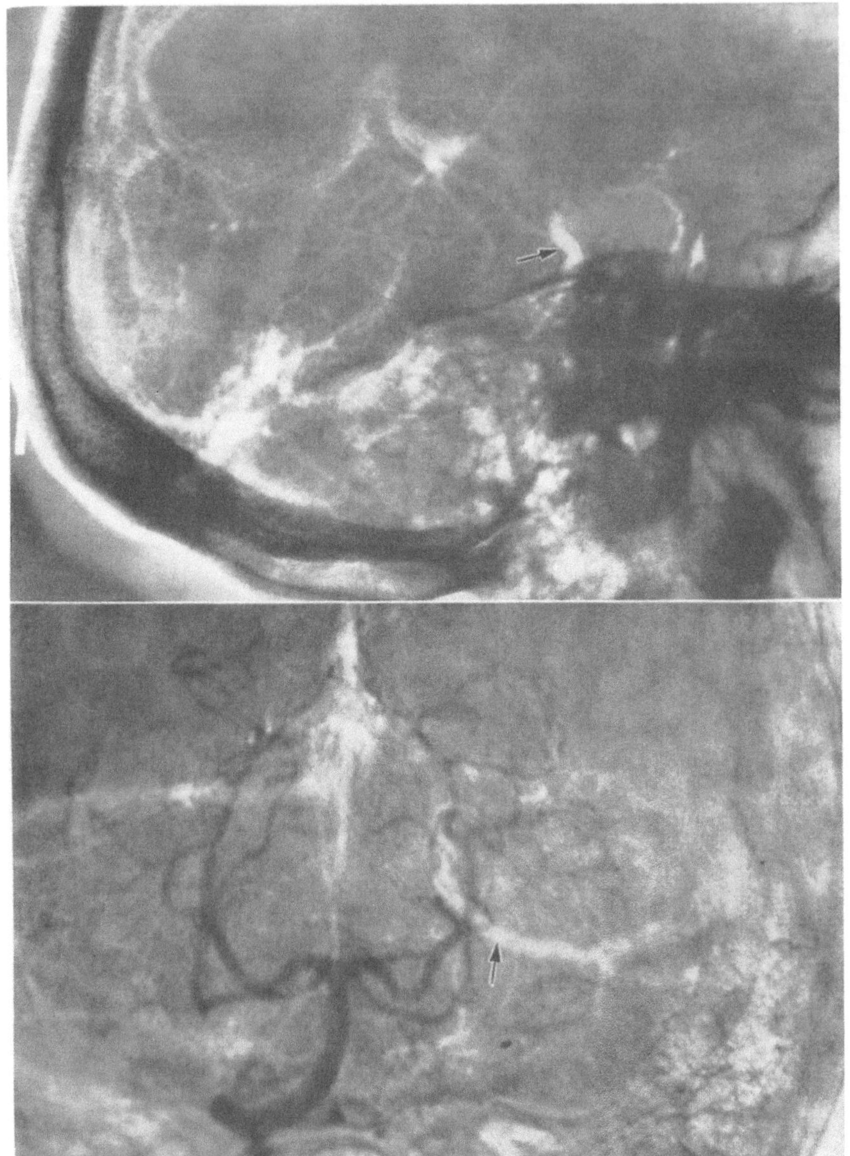

Fig. 61a
Dilatation of the petrosal vein which joins the mesencephalic vein

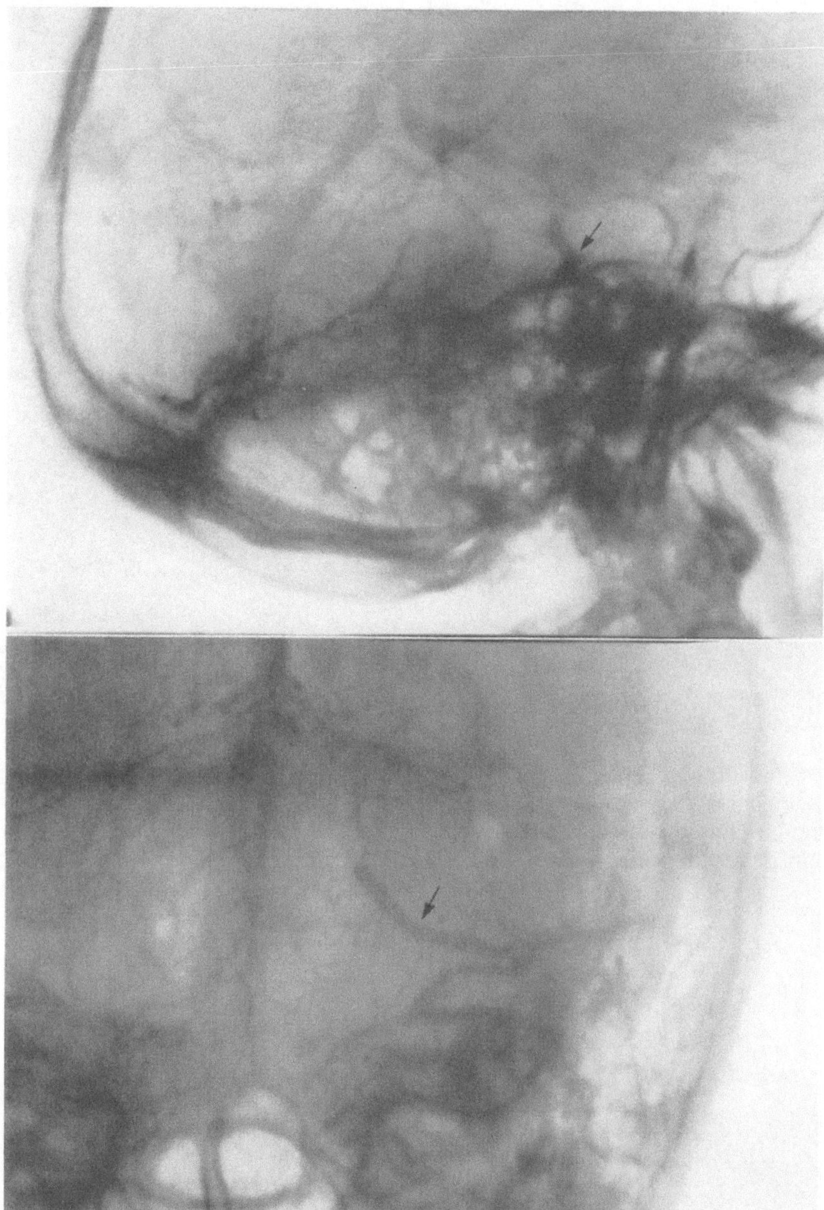

Fig. 61 b

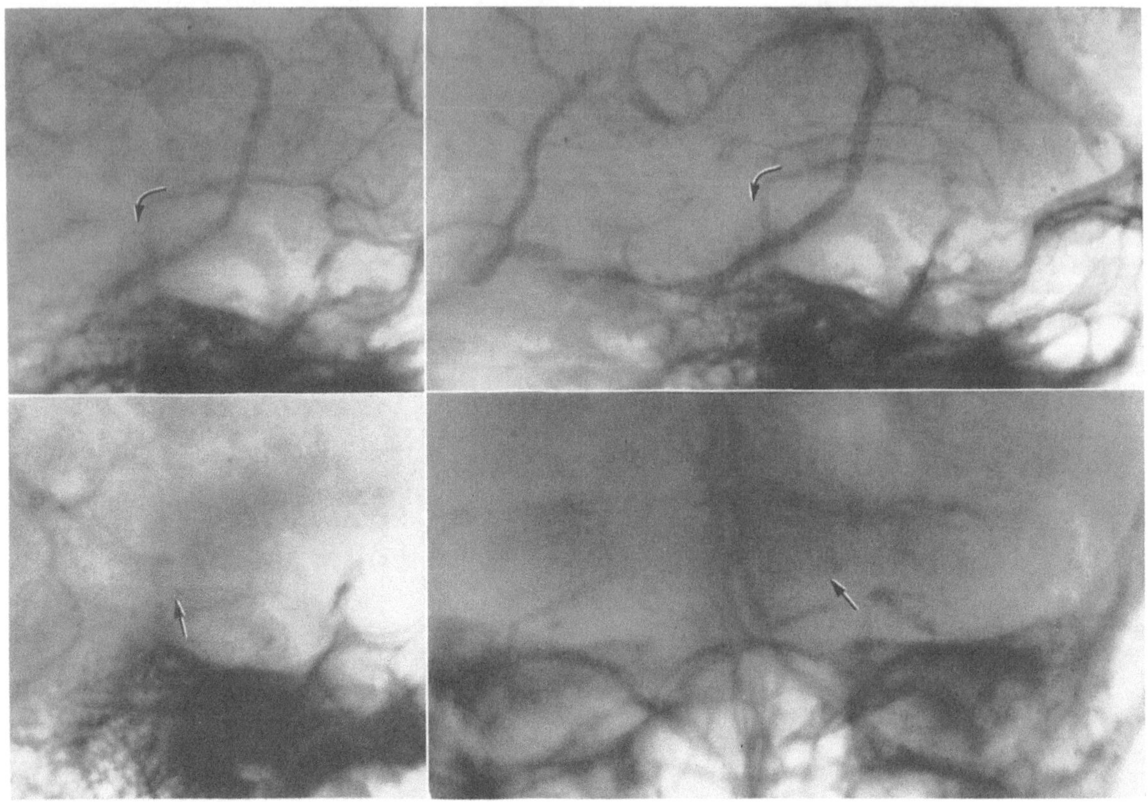

Fig. 62. Lateral mesencephalic vein. *Top :* The vein is opacified in carotid angiography. *Bottom :* The vein is also opacified in vertebral angiography

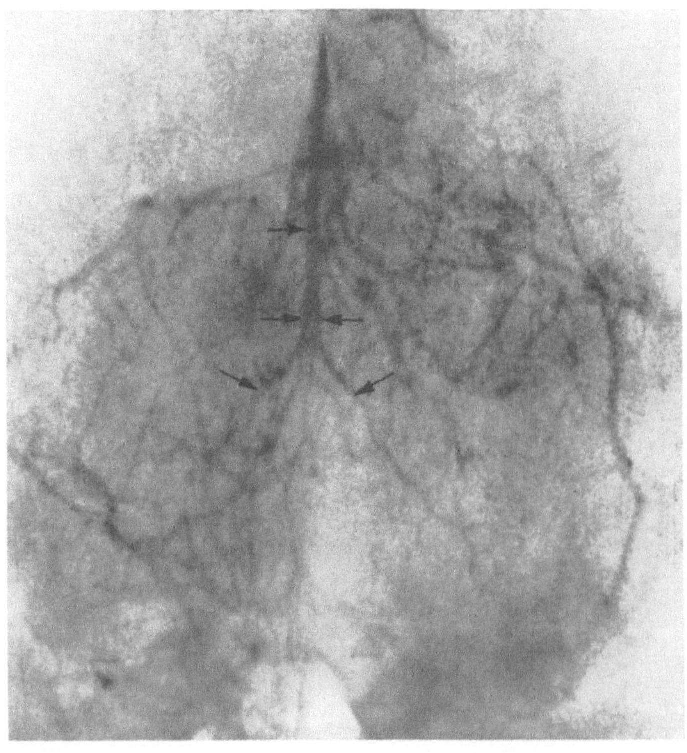

Fig. 63a

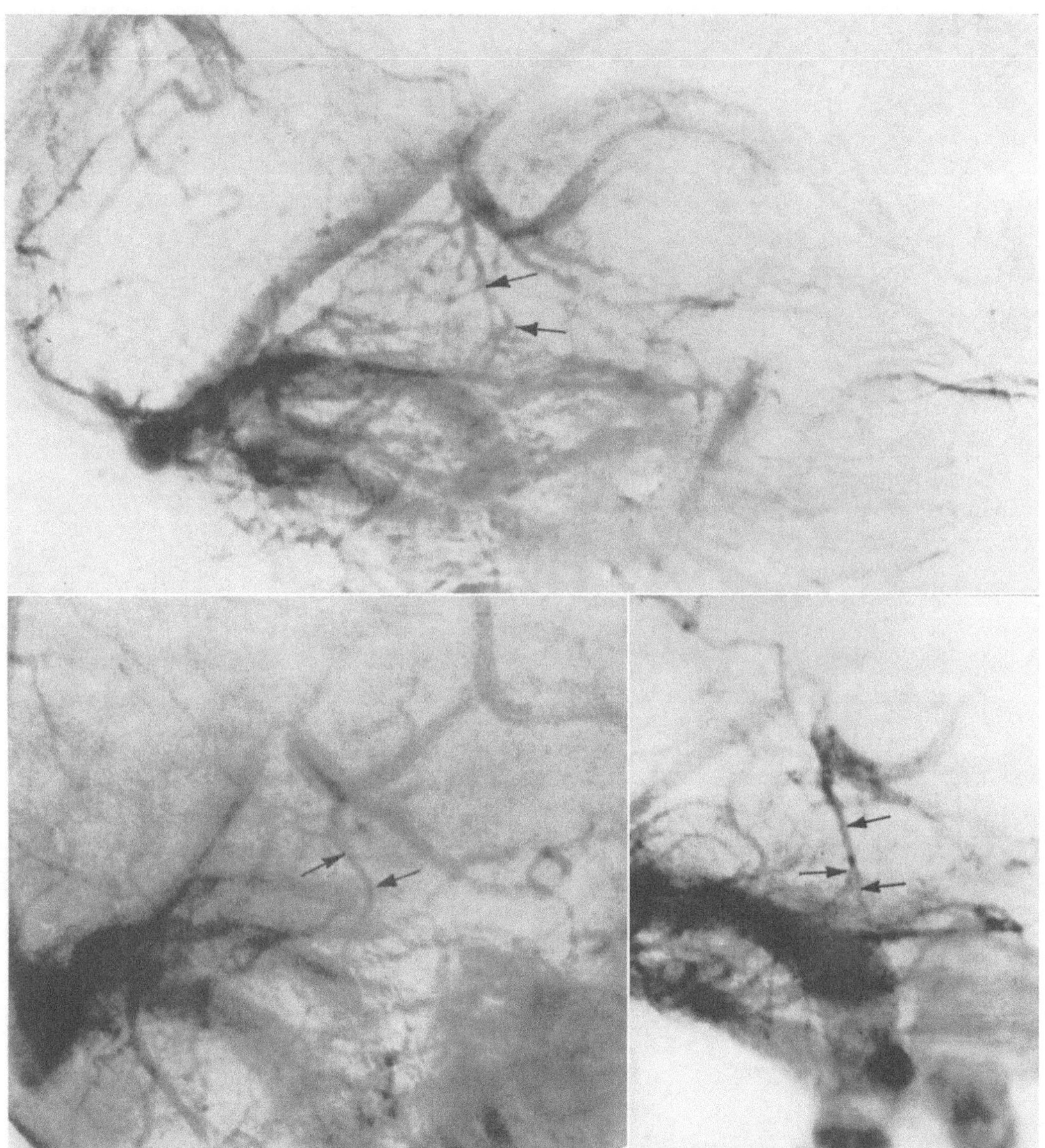

Fig. 63b

Fig. 63a and b
Precentral vein and variants

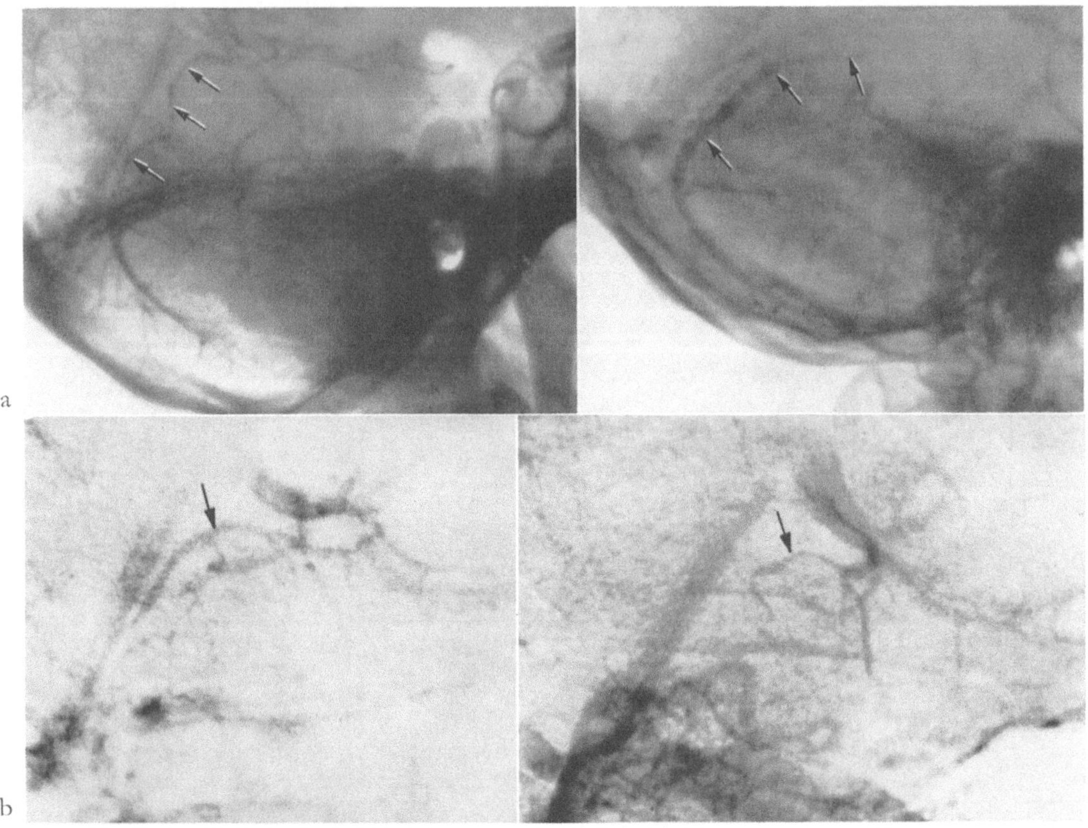

a

b

Fig. 64a and b
Superior vermian vein
and variants

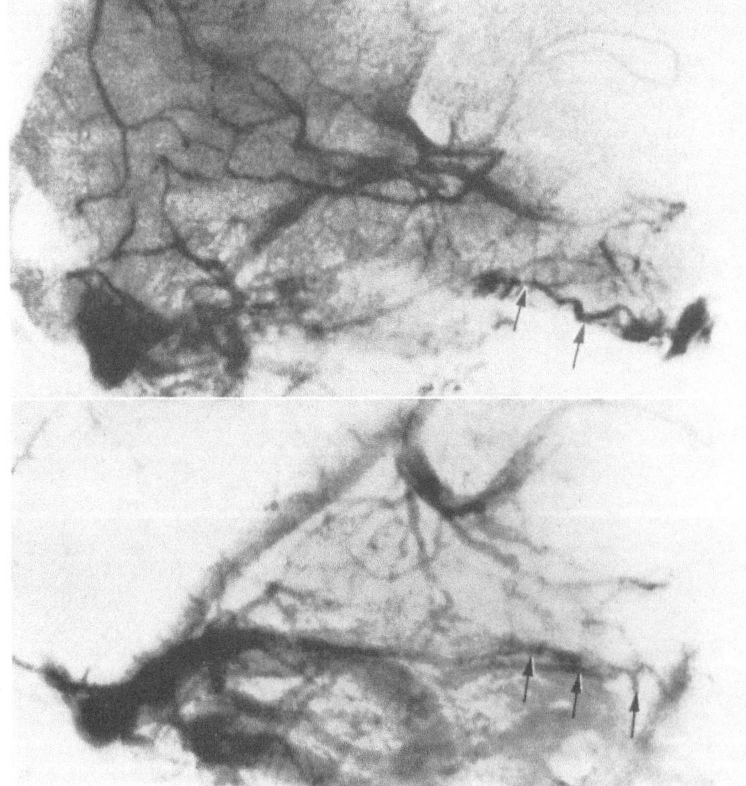

Fig. 65
Tentorial veins

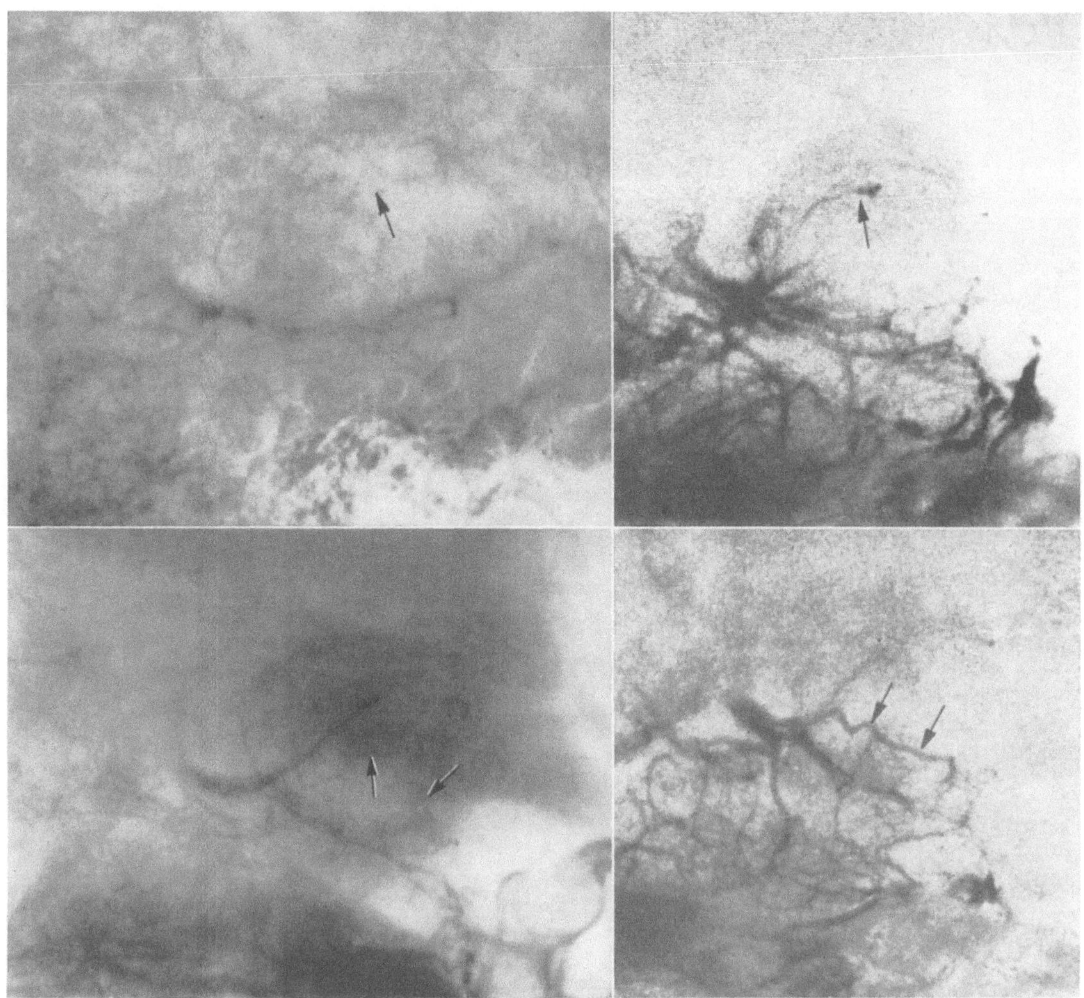

Fig. 66
Thalamic veins

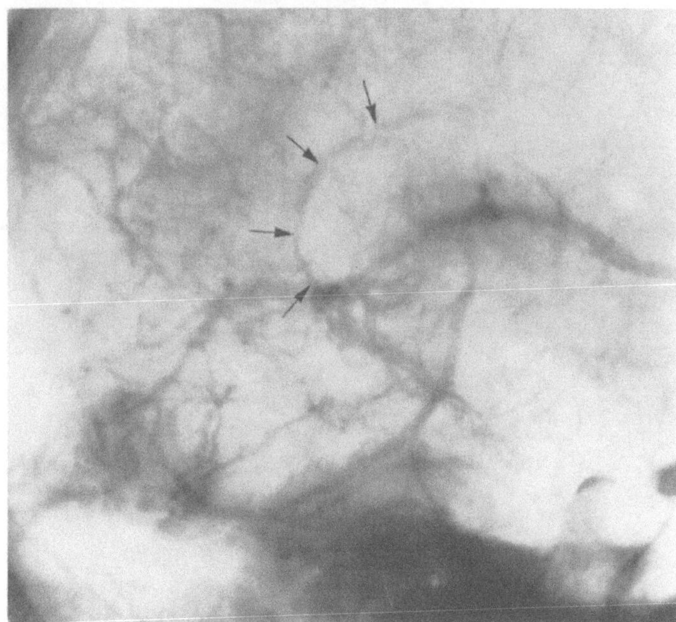

Fig. 67
Posterior pericallosal vein

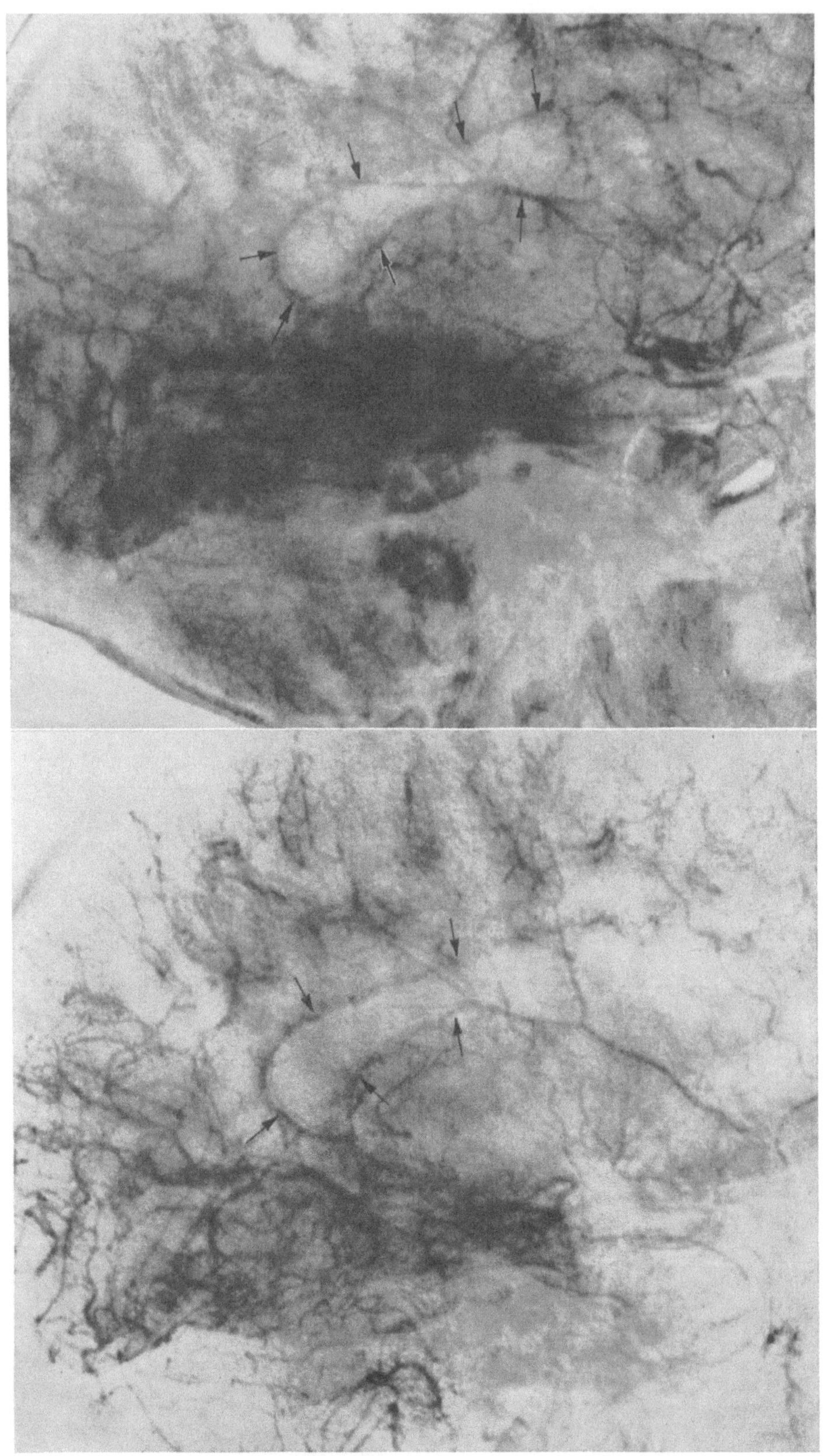

Fig. 68. Normal appearance of the splenium

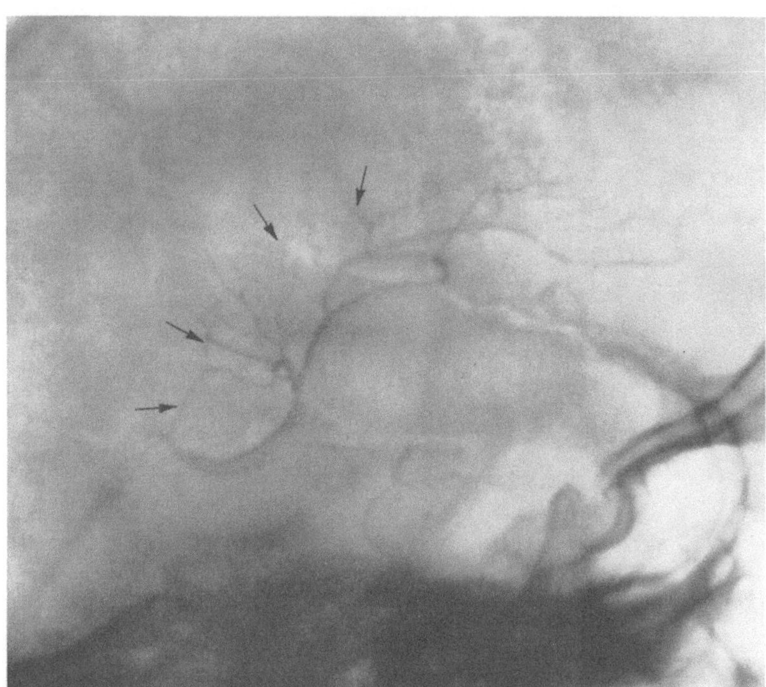

Fig. 69
Ventricular veins joining
the internal cerebral vein

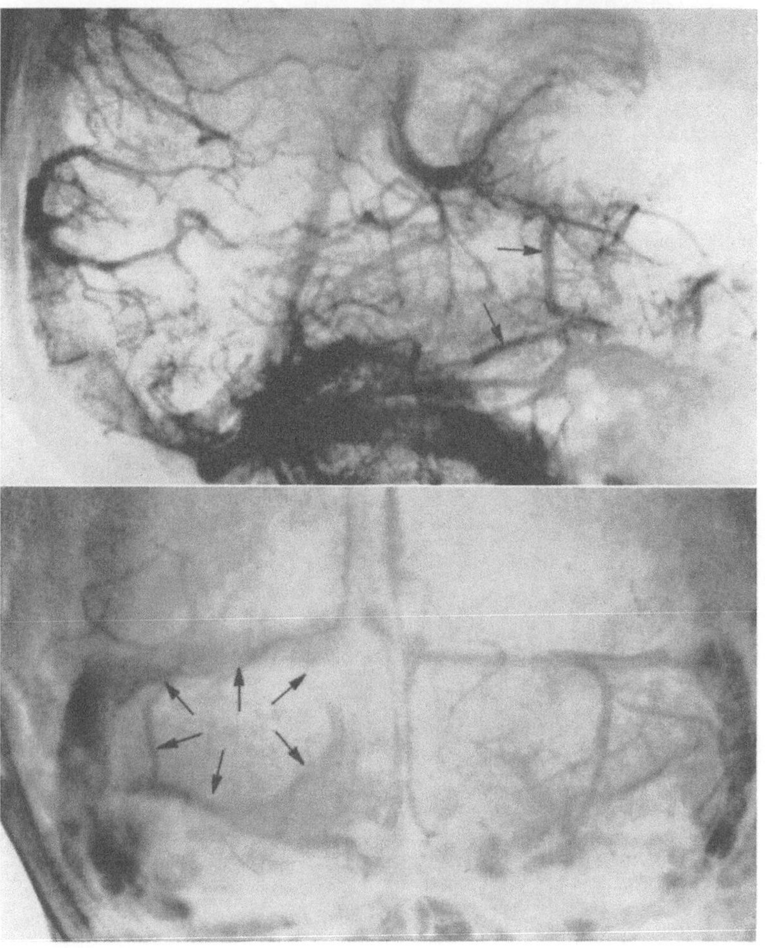

Fig. 70
Cerebellar-mesencephalic
venous circle

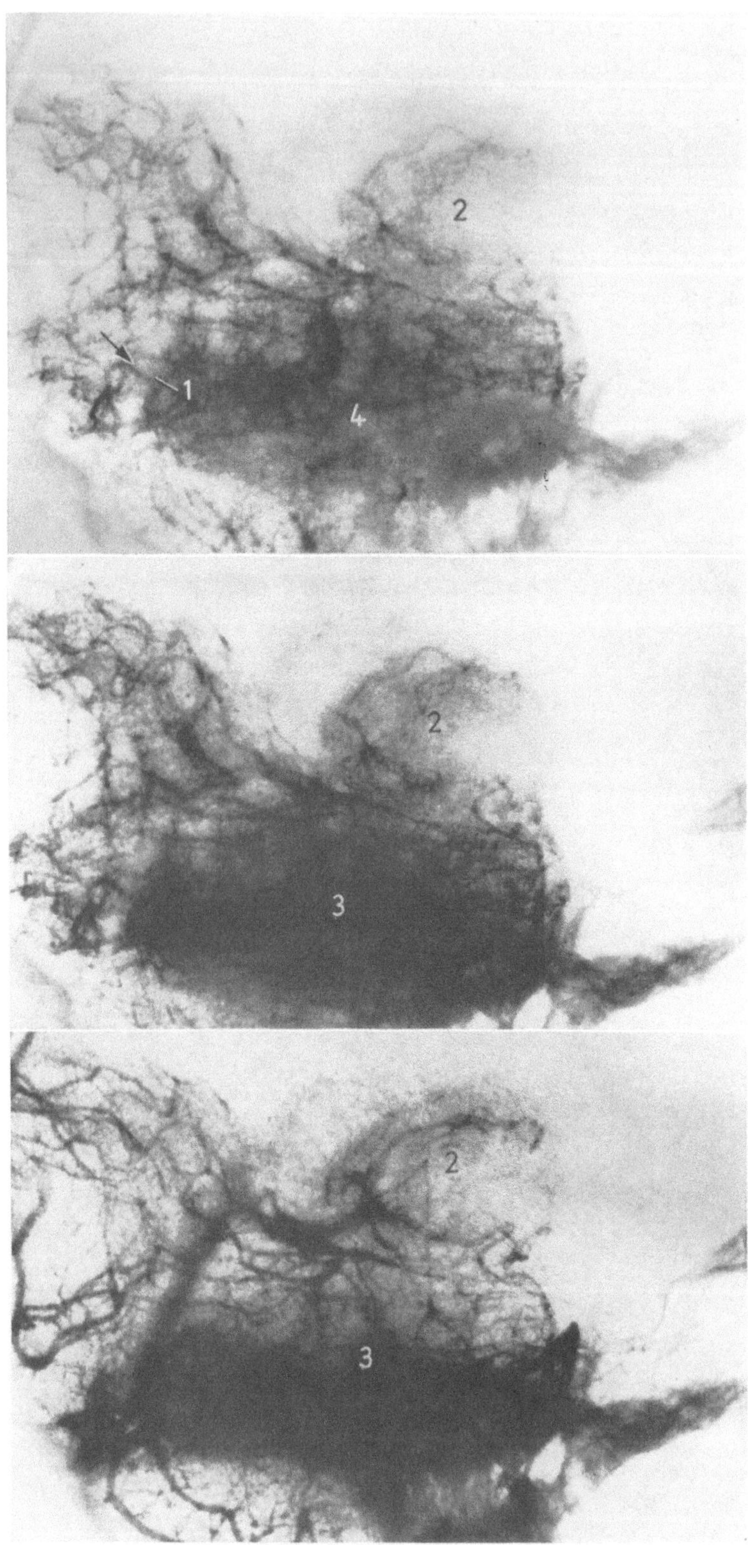

Fig. 71
Capillarography of the thalamic region: *1* Avascular zone of the tentorium.
2 Venous capillarography in the thalamic region. *3* Capillarography in the posterior fossa. *4* Area of the IVth ventricle

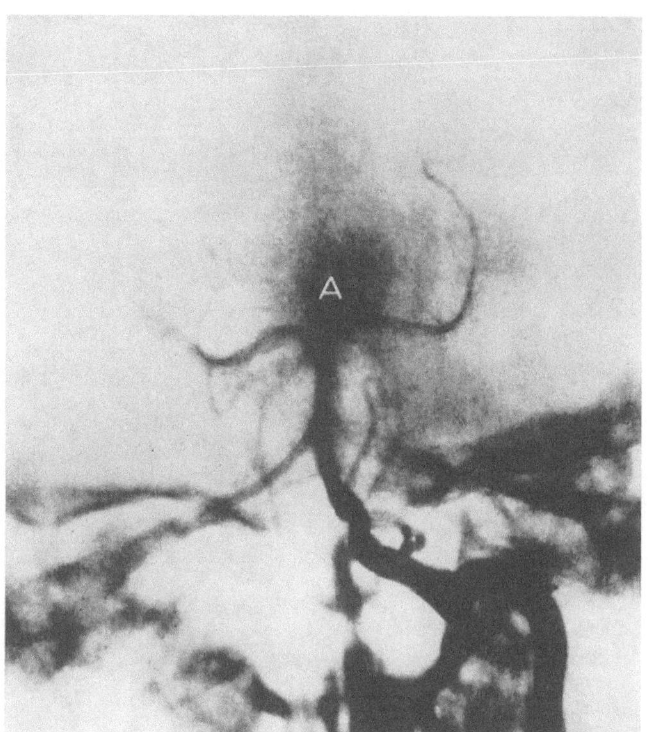

Fig. 72
Artefact of the technique of substraction (*A*)

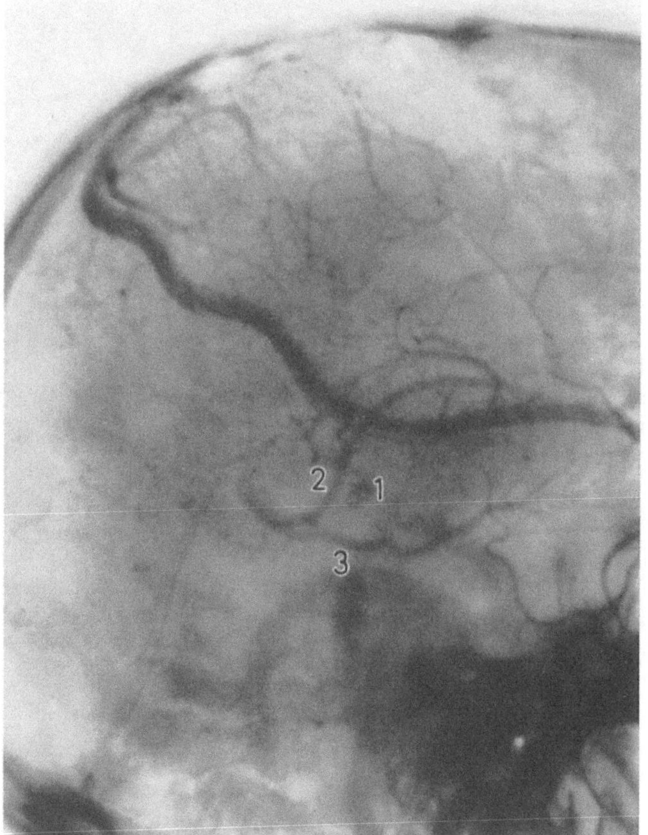

Fig. 73
Topographic relation between the calcified pineal gland and the veins:
1 Pineal gland. *2* Internal cerebral vein. *3* Basal vein

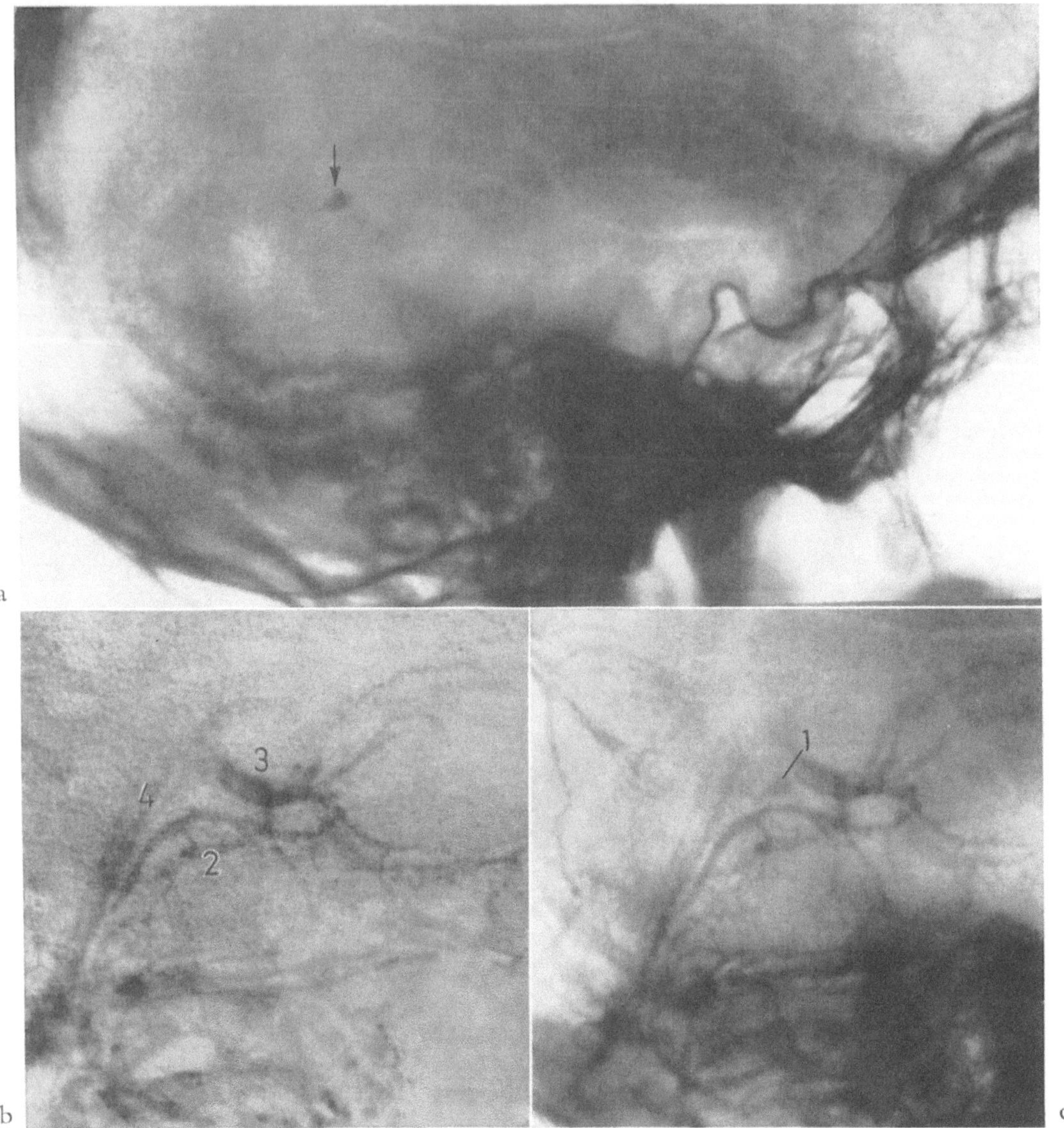

Fig. 74a–c
a) Visible calcification on standard film. b and c) Phlebography permits to localise this calcification in the superior vermian cistern. *1* Calcification. *2* Superior vermian vein. *3* Great vein of Galen. *4* Straight sinus

Fig. 75
Venous topogram:
S Splenium
Th Thalamus
CI Cisterna
interpeduncularis
CP Cisterna pontis
P Peduncle
M Mesencephalon
V Vermis
svv superior
vermian vein
bv basal vein
ipv interpeduncular
vein
pmv ponto-mesen-
cephalic vein
lmv lateral mesen-
cephalic vein
pv precentral vein

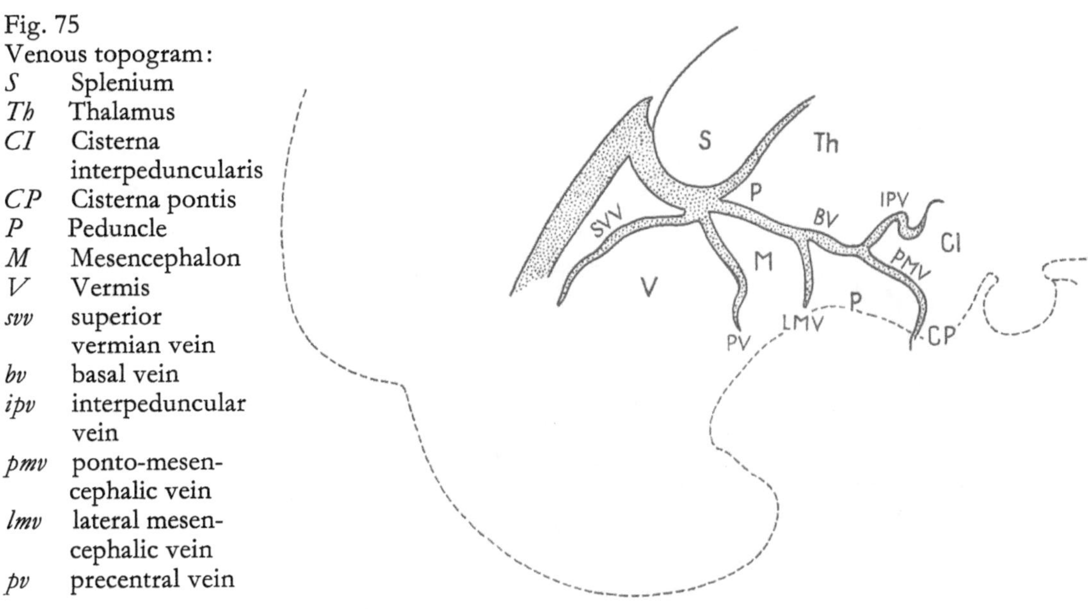

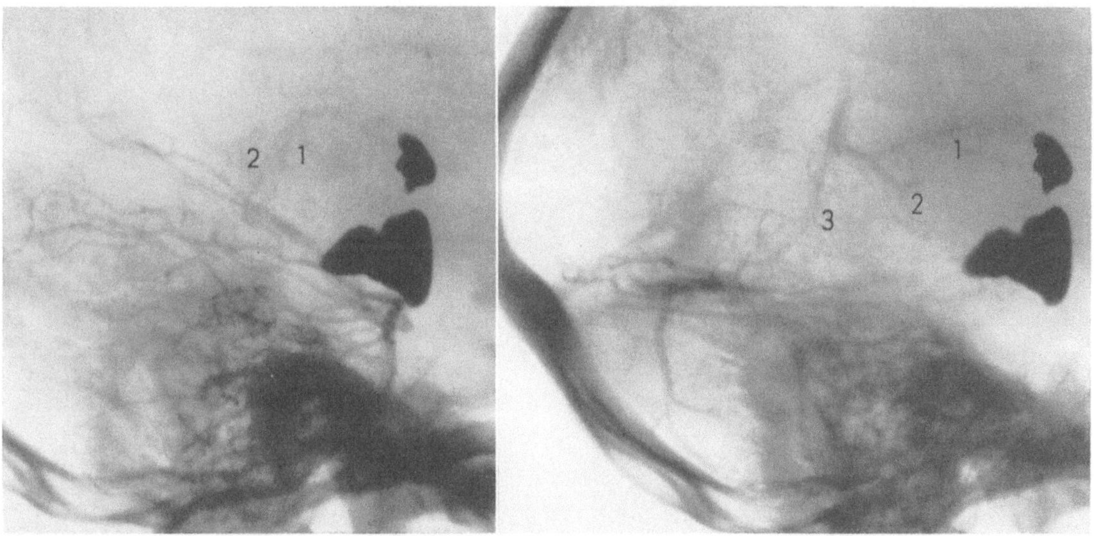

Fig. 76
Pinealoma in a woman 43 years of age which presents a sign of Parinaud, a bilateral sign of Babinski and a meningeal and confusional syndrome. Pantopaque ventriculography shows important bulging and forward displacements of the posterior wall of the IIIrd ventricle. Owing to simultaneous visualization of arterial and venous vessels, the tumour can be entirely outlined. *Figure to the left : arterial phase.* The displacement backwards and upwards of the posterior choroidal arteries is more particularly marked by the postero-medial choroidal artery. *1* Postero-medial choroidal artery. *2* Postero-lateral choroidal artery. *Figure to the right : venous phase. 1* A hypertrophied superior thalamic vein straddling the upper area of the tumour. *2* A hypertrophic vein draining the posterior region of the tumour towards the great vein of Galen. *3* Basal vein displaced backwards and upwards. (Venous hammock)

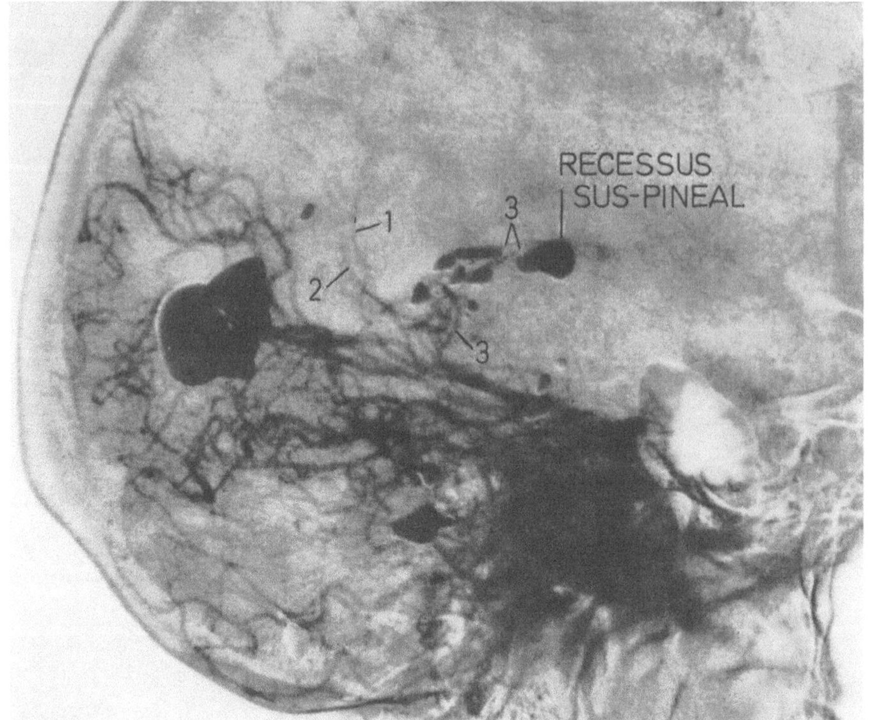

Fig. 77a

Fig. 77a–d
A woman 53 years of age, admitted for a confusional syndrome, suffering from a pinealoma checked anatomically. As in the preceding case, pantopaque ventriculography complements usefully angiography. The sub-pineal recess outlines the antero-superior pole of the tumour (a). *1* The posterior pericallosal artery, slightly displaced backwards, presents a practically normal pathological picture. *2* The postero-lateral choroidal artery, markedly displaced backwards, crosses the course of the pericallosal artery and thus confirms the thalamo-peduncular extension of the tumour. *3* The posteromedial choroidal arteries are hypertrophic and displaced backwards and upwards, but retain nonetheless a "3"-shaped configuration. The direction taken by these displacements results from the fact that the arteries are embodied in the tumour. b) Anterior aspect in the cross section of the tumour. c) Anterior aspect in the cross section at the level of the cerebral peduncles. d) Posterior aspect of the preceding cross section. Note the asymmetrical development of the tumour

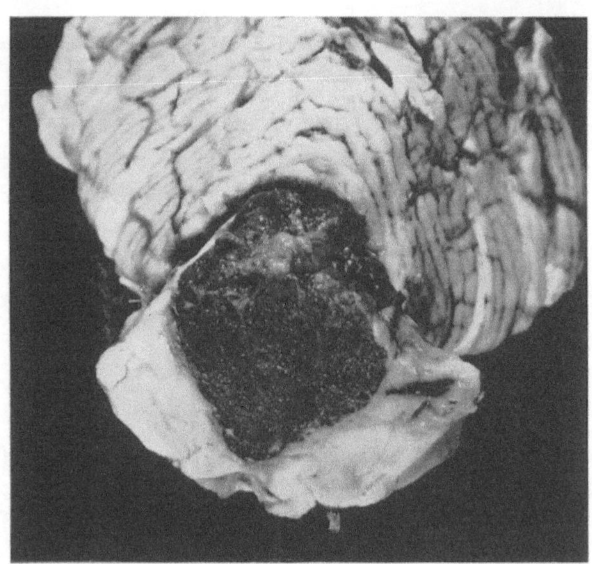

Fig. 77b

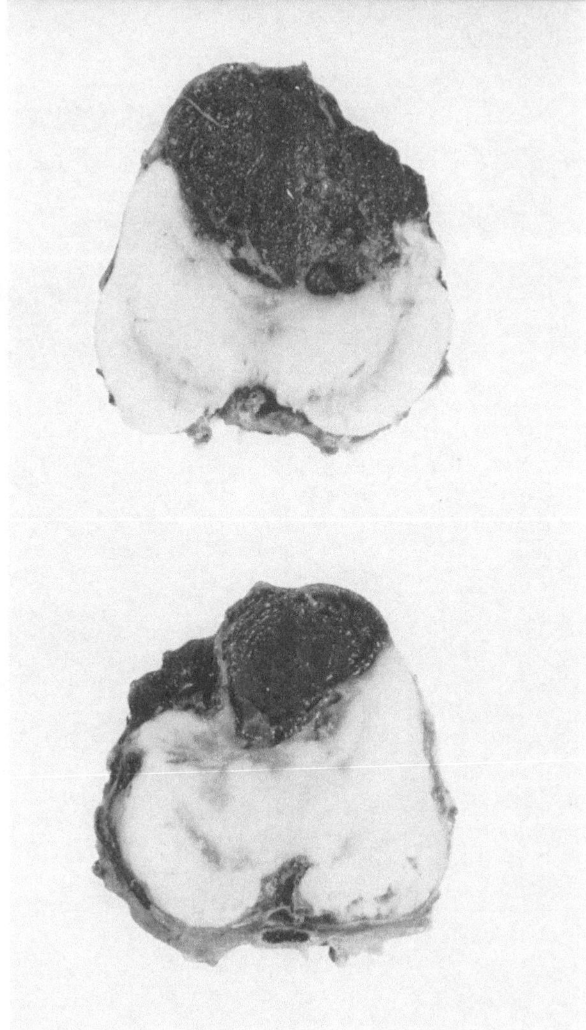

Fig. 77c

Fig. 77d

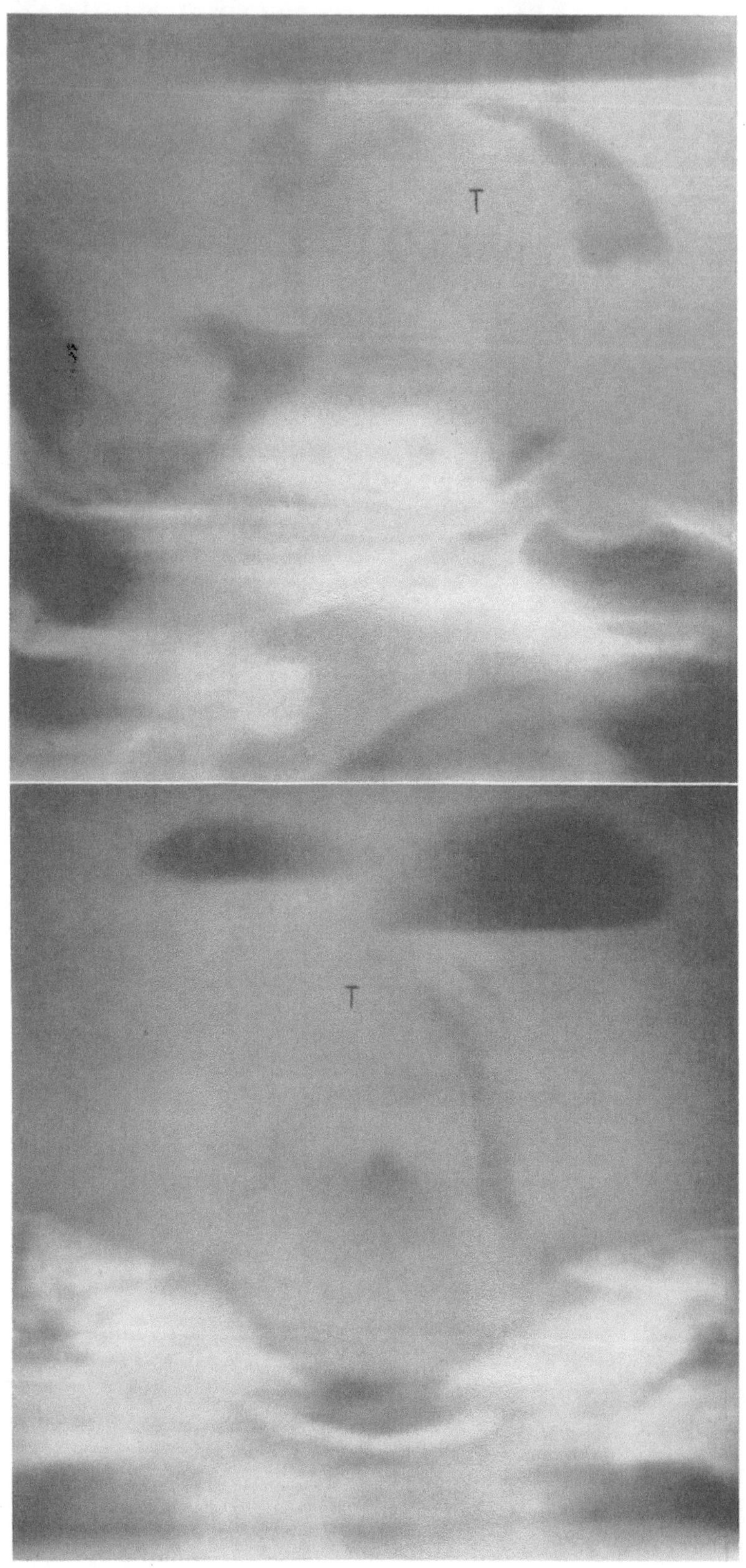

Fig. 78a
Legend see p. 104

Fig. 78b

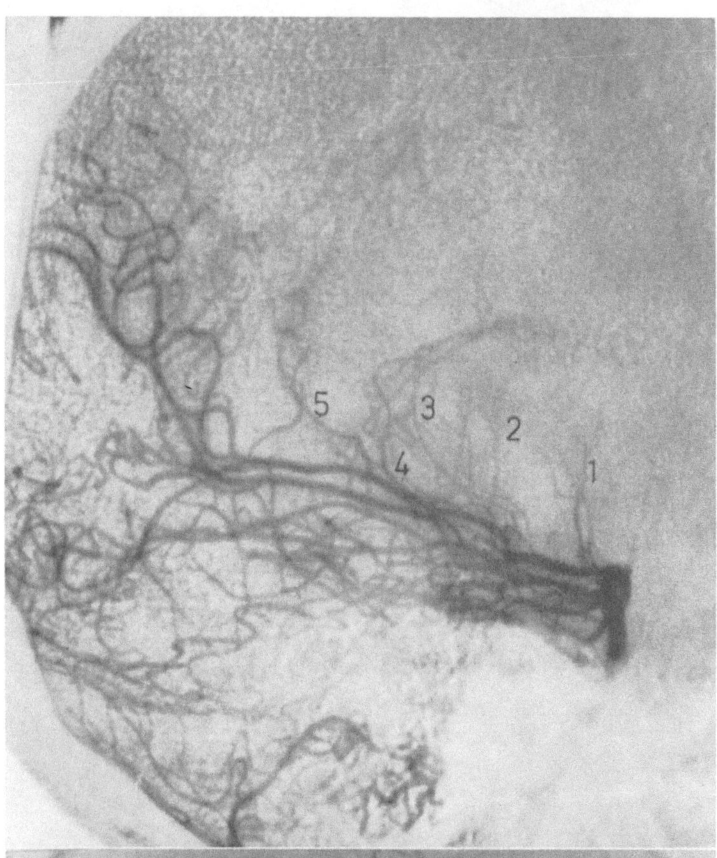

Fig. 78d

Fig. 78c

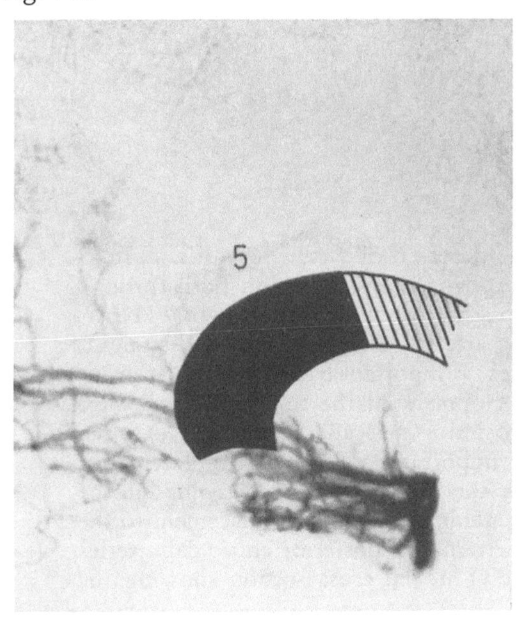

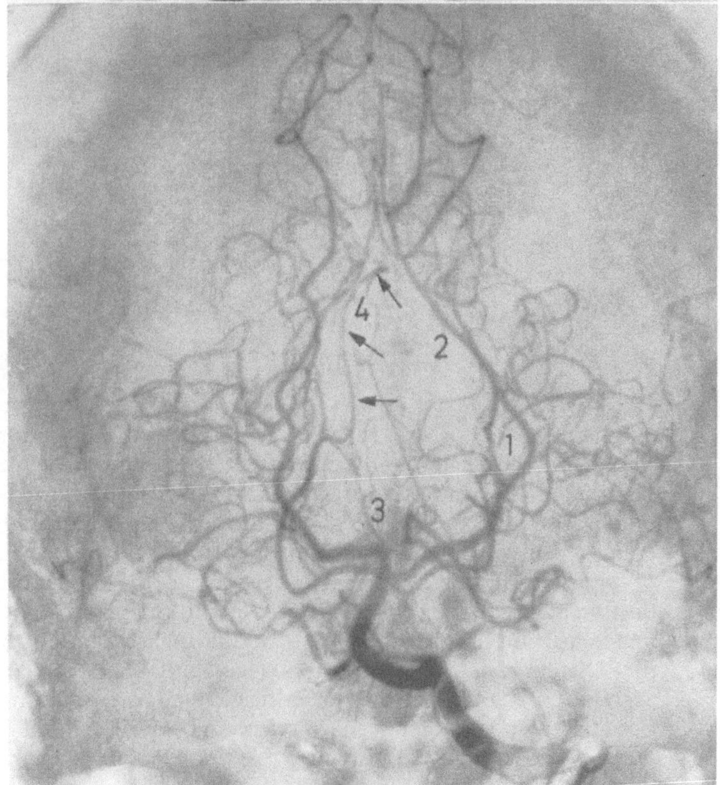

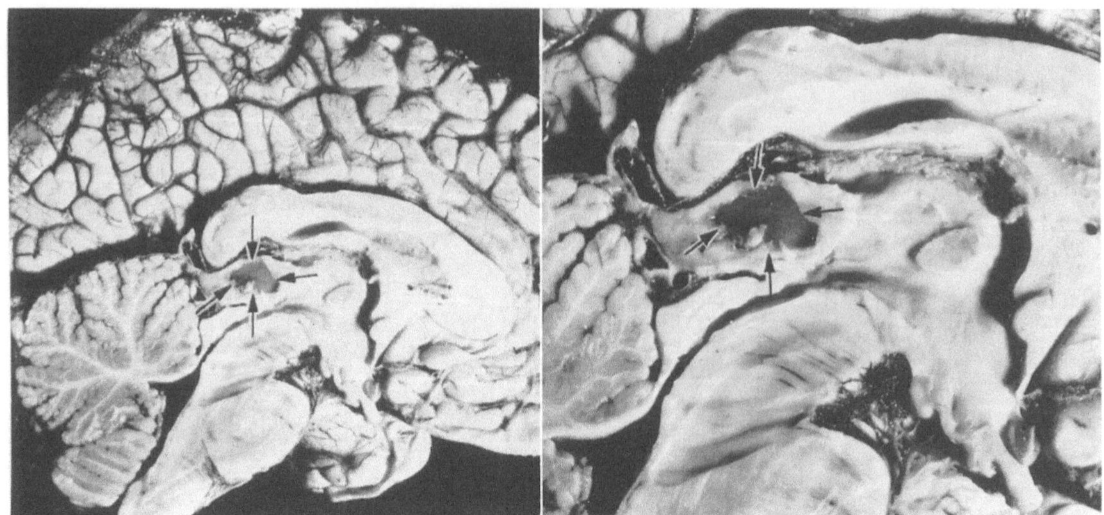

Fig. 78e   f

Fig. 78a–f
Woman 24 years of age, suffering from a pineal astrocytoma, deceased of virous hepatitis. a) Fractional gas encephalography permitting to localise a mesencephalic mass expansion both through ventricular deformities and the characteristic backward displacement of the cisterns, b) *1* Hypertrophy and straightening of the posterior thalamo-perforating arteries. *2* Hypertrophy and straightening of the colliculi quadrigemini et corpori geniculati arteries. *3* Important backward displacement of a postero-medial choroidal artery due to the medial development of the tumour. *4* Backward displacement of the postero-lateral choroidal arteries. *5* Posterior pericallosal arteries. c) Superimposition of Löfgren's diagram permitting to outline the importance of arterial displacements. d) *1* Displacement of the posterior cerebral artery towards the exterior. *2* Straightening of the pretentorial segment of the posterior cerebral artery. *3* Straightening and slight displacement to the right of the posterior thalamo-perforating arteries. *4* The surrounding posterior choroidal arteries outline the rounded contours of the tumour (arrow). e and f) Medial cross section showing the tumour: cystic astrocytoma of the pineal body

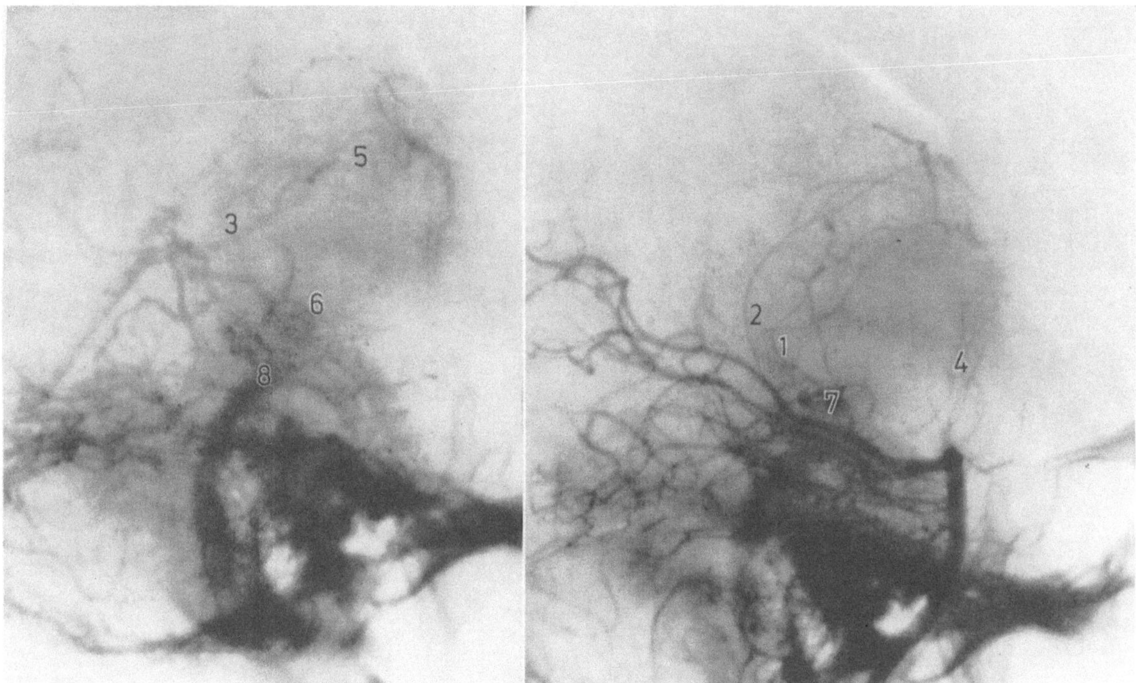

Fig. 79
A very important pineal mass which invades the splenium, the thalamus and the peduncle. The expansion of the pineal mass is placed in evidence by the increase in curvature of the postero-medial (*1*) and postero-lateral (*2*) choroidal arteries. Due to venous alterations in front of the right sinus (*3*) an invasion of the splenium is recognizable. Alterations of the posterior thalamo-perforating arteries (*4*), of the internal cerebral vein (*5*) and of the terminal segment of the basal vein (*6*) point out the invasion of the thalamus. Peduncular invasion is suspected in the following anomalies: -pathological vessels above the first curvature of the posterior cerebral artery (*7*), -abnormal veins forming a complex network in the region of the precentral and lateral mesencephalic veins (*8*)

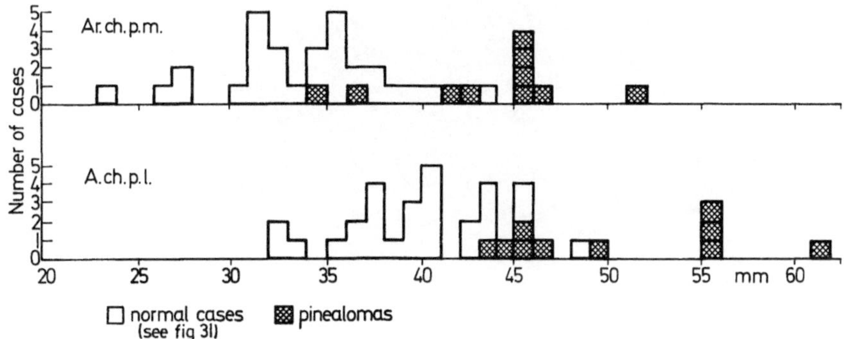

Fig. 80
The distance between the postero-lateral and medial choroidal arteries with relation to the upper extremity of the basilar trunk in 10 cases of pinealoma. Note the shifting to the right of the measured values in cases of pinealoma

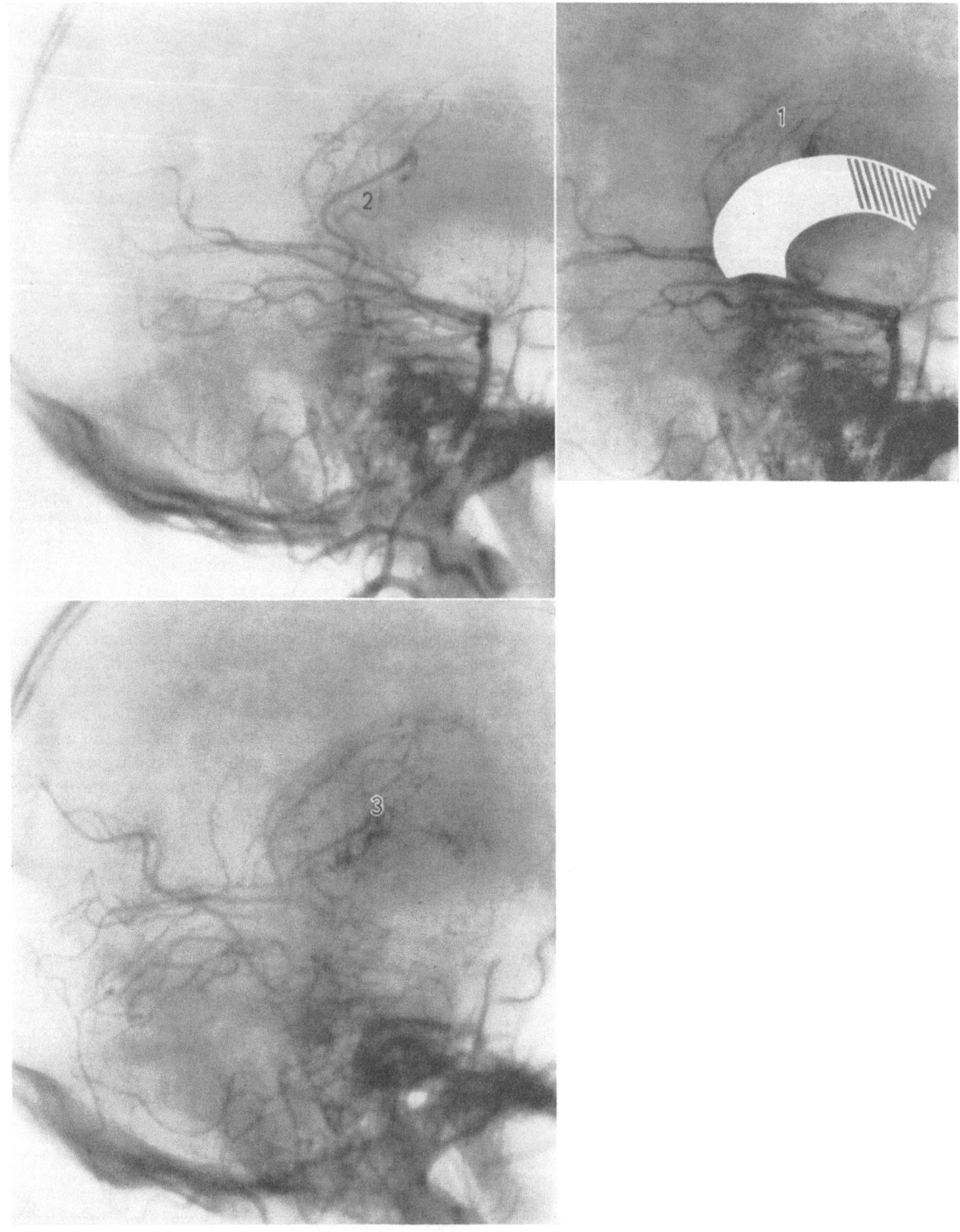

Fig. 81
Tumour of the pineal gland. *1* Important arterial displacement characterised by a falling out of the arterial diagram. *2* Considerable hypertrophy in the diameter of the posterior choroidal arteries. *3* Numerous pathological vessels pointing out the malignant nature of the tumour

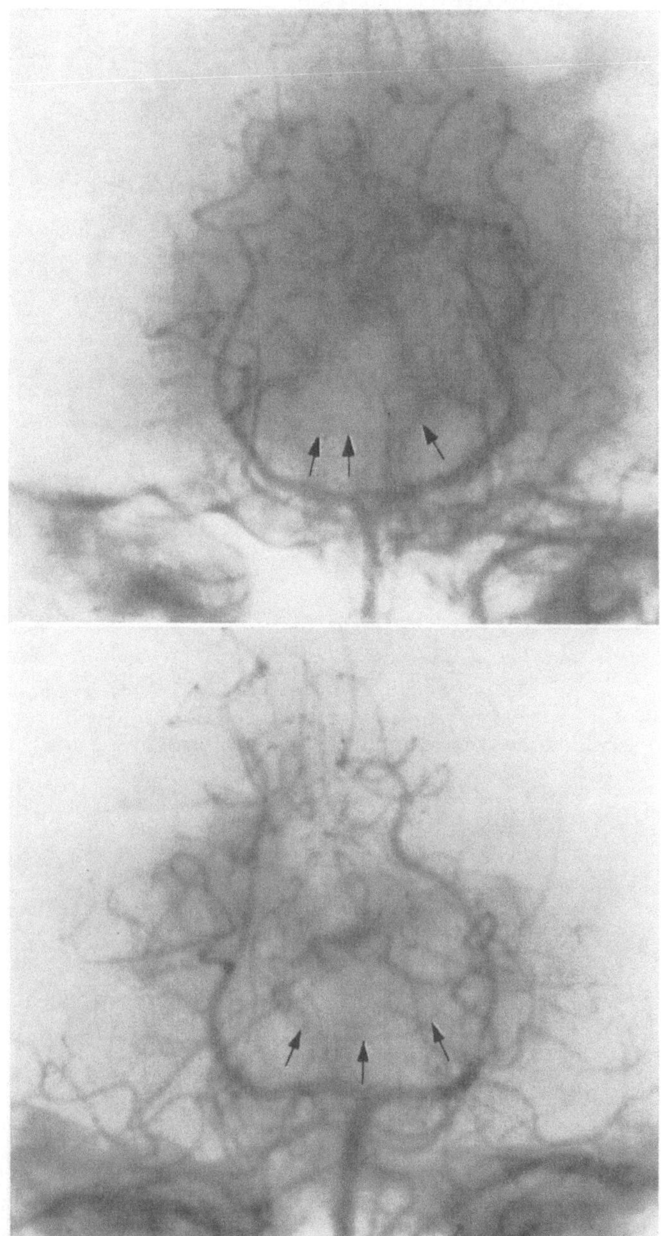

Fig. 82
Arterial hammock in two cases of pinealoma (see fig. 25)

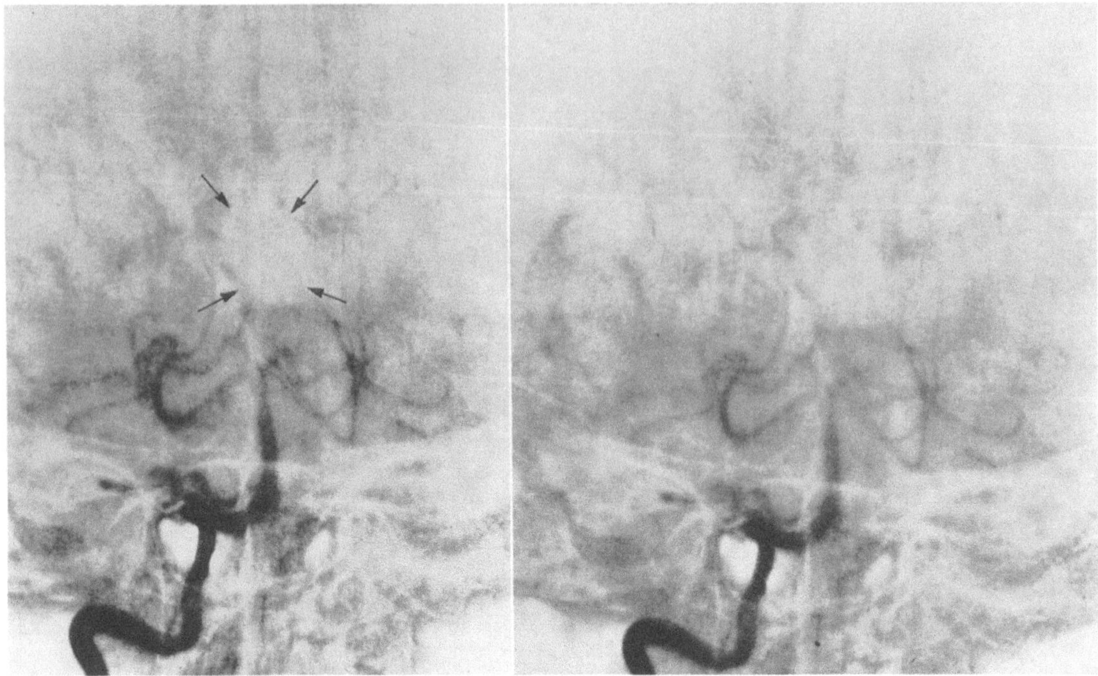

Fig. 83
Avascular zone corresponding to a pinealoma

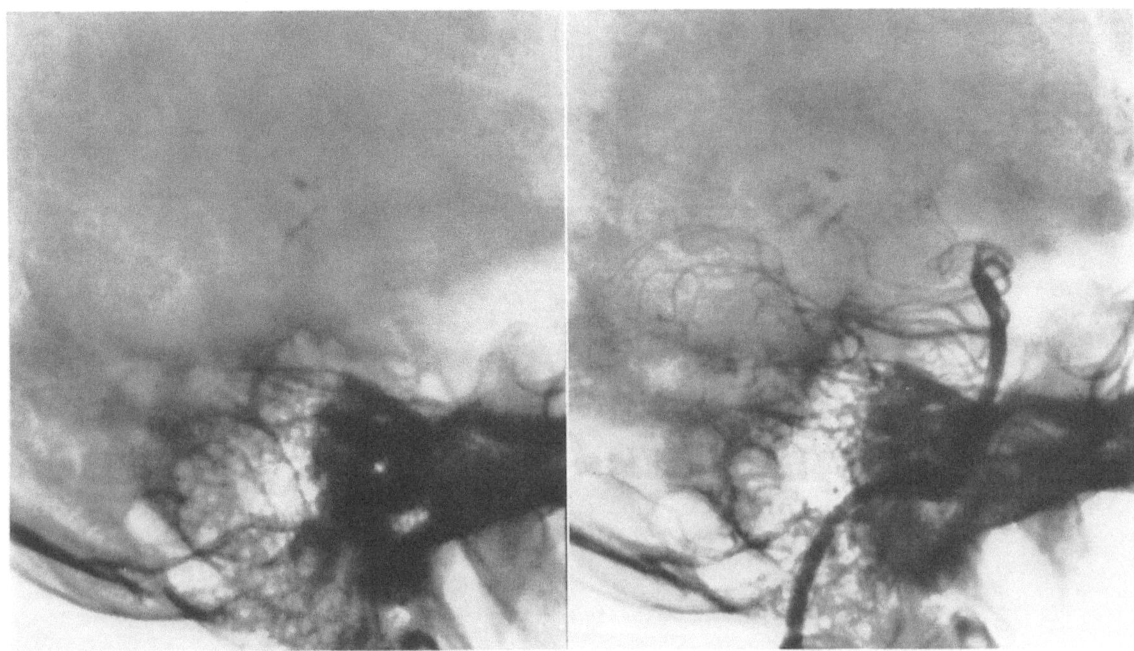

Fig. 84
Dislocation of the posterior choroidal arteries in the area occupied by the calcifications of a pinealoma

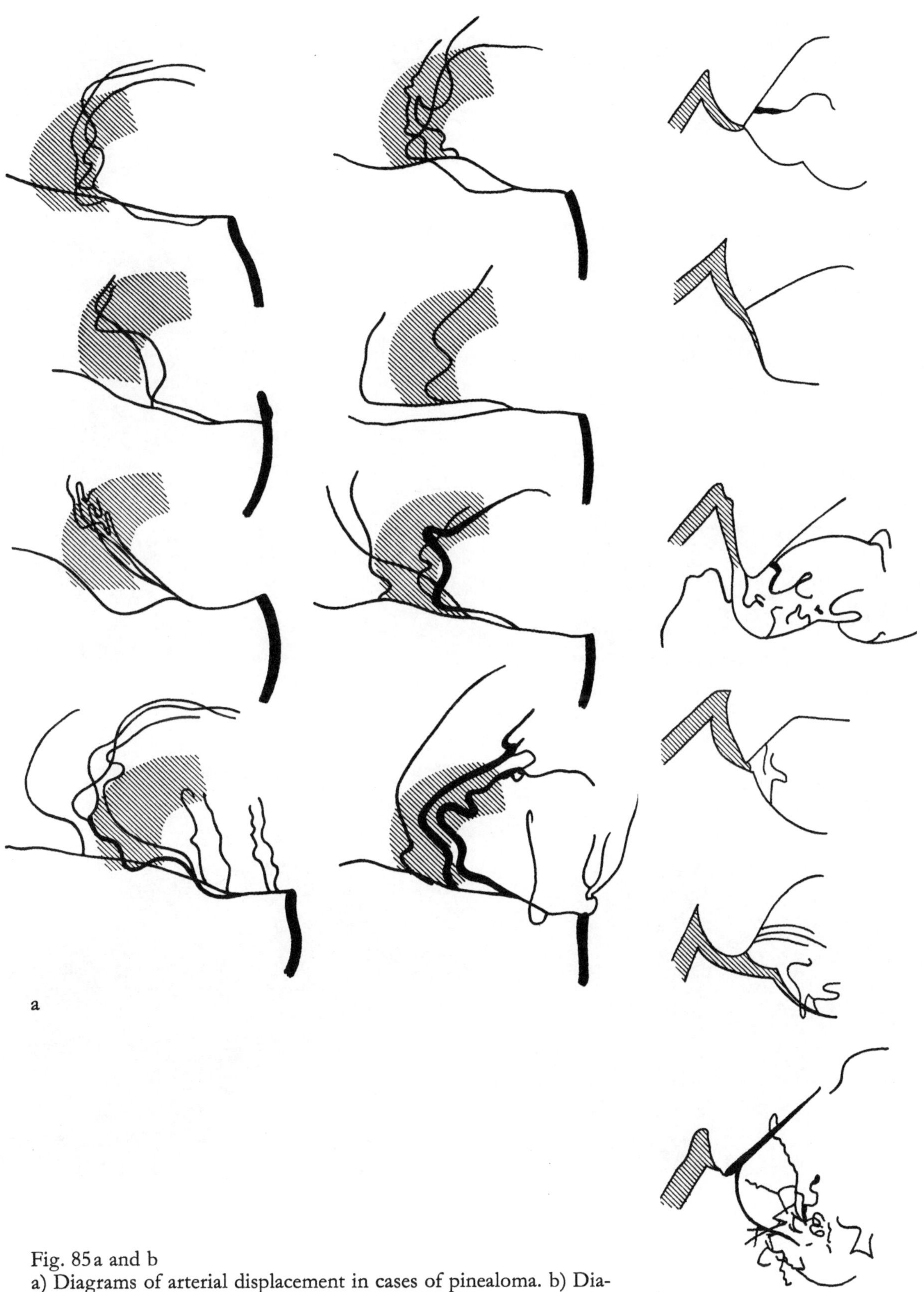

Fig. 85a and b
a) Diagrams of arterial displacement in cases of pinealoma. b) Diagrams of venous alterations in cases of pinealoma

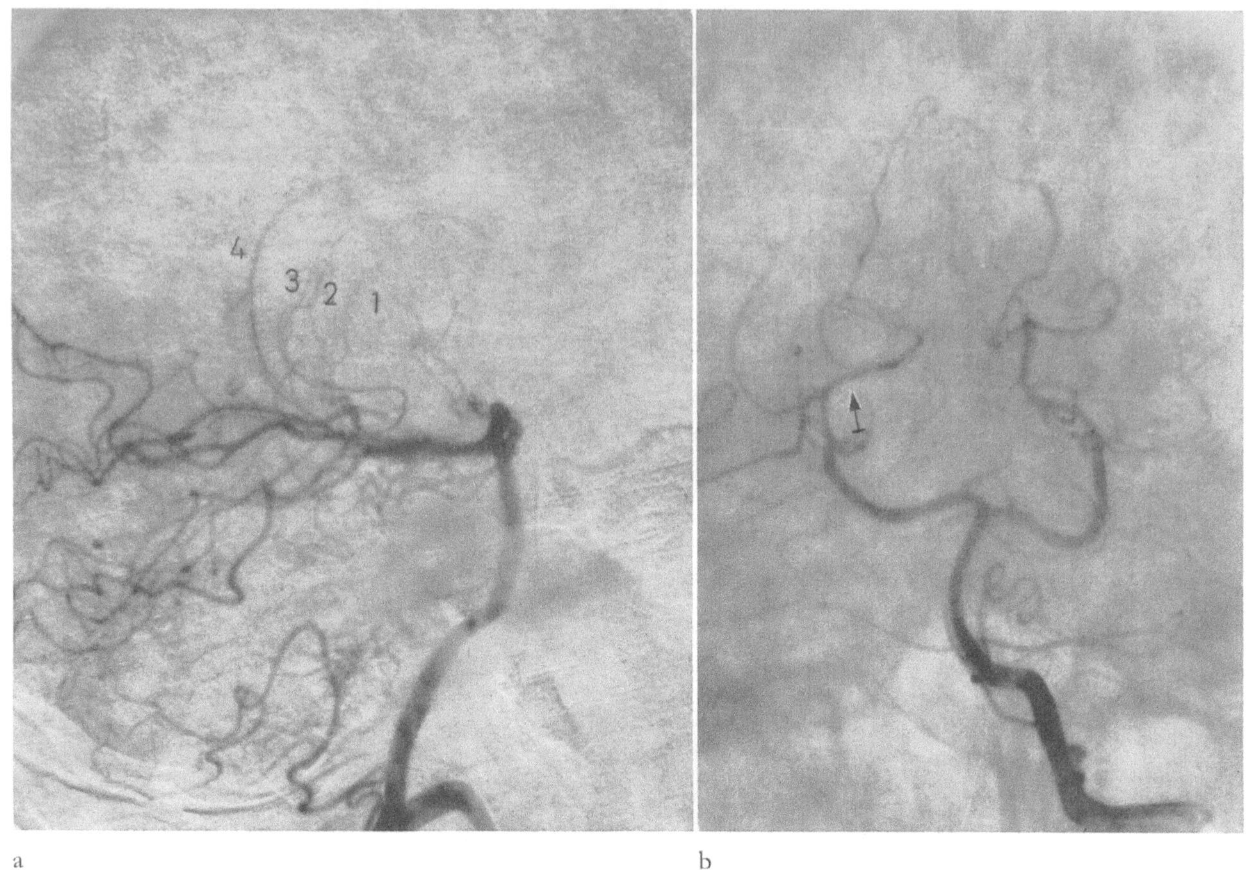

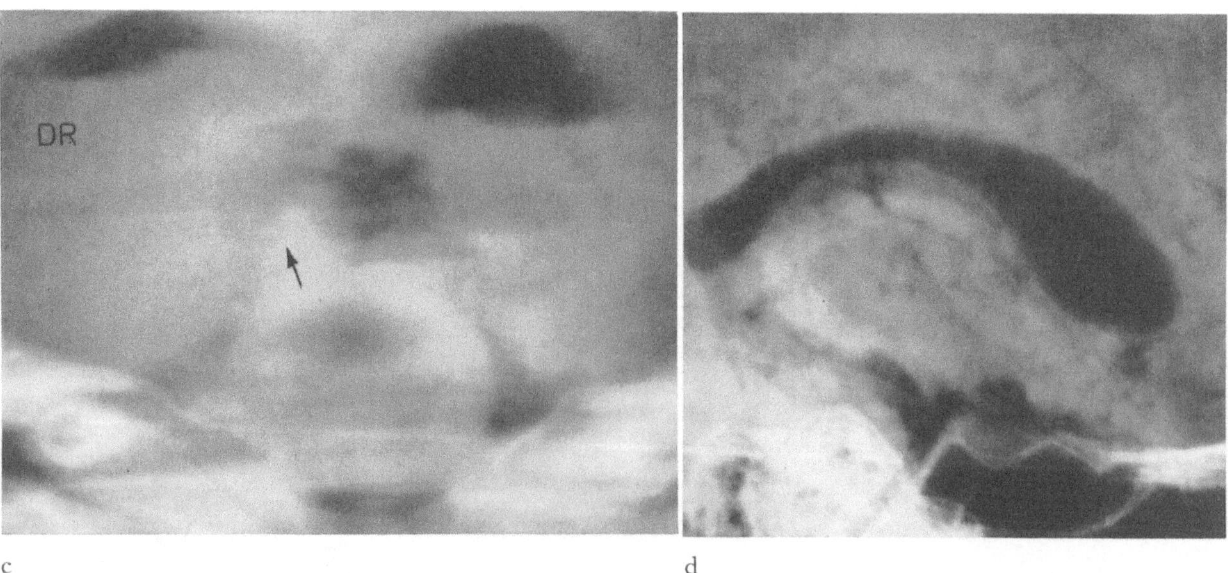

Fig. 86a–d

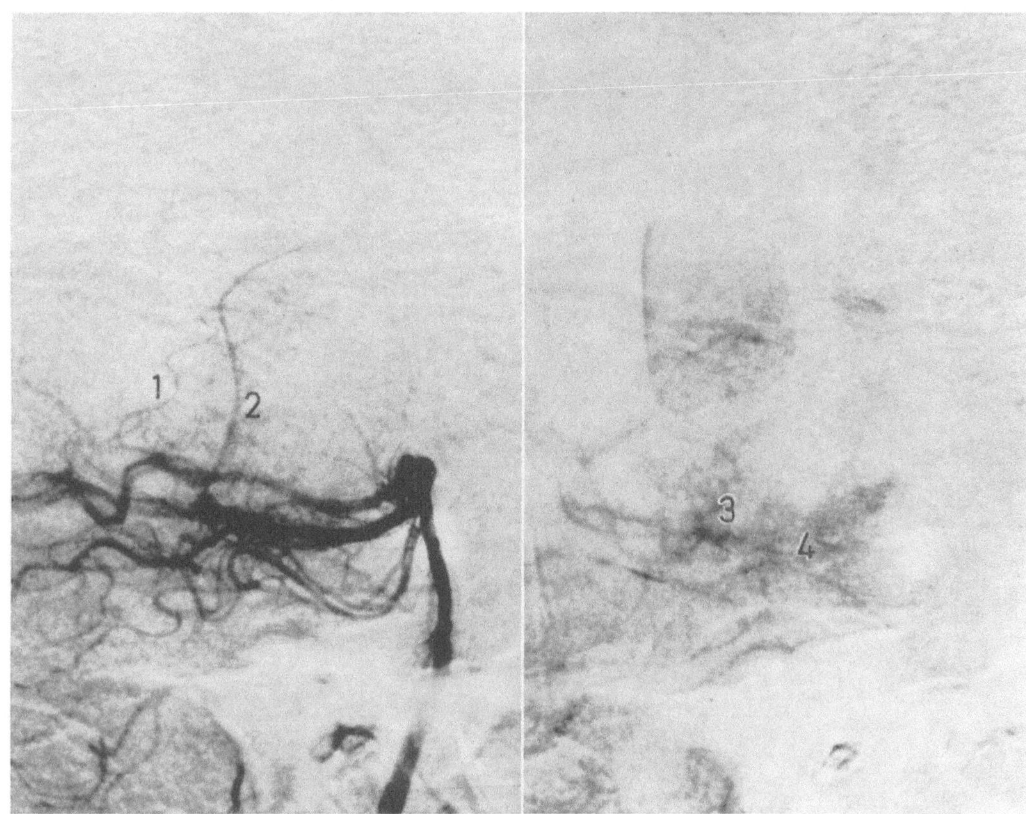

Fig. 87
Posterior thalamic tumour. *1* Postero-medial choroidal artery in a normal position. *2* Postero-lateral choroidal artery embodied in the tumour. It is deformed and rigid, its course is convex forwards. *3* Dilated and irregular thalamic veins. *4* Tumoral capillarography

Fig. 86a–d
Thalamo-peduncular tumour. a) *1* and *2* postero-medial and lateral choroidal arteries not displaced on the healthy side. *3* and *4* the same arteries are markedly displaced on the tumoral side. b) Deviation of the posterior cerebral artery by the tumoral expansion (↑). c) Invasion of the quadrigeminal plate (↑). d) Elevation of the floor of the lateral ventricle

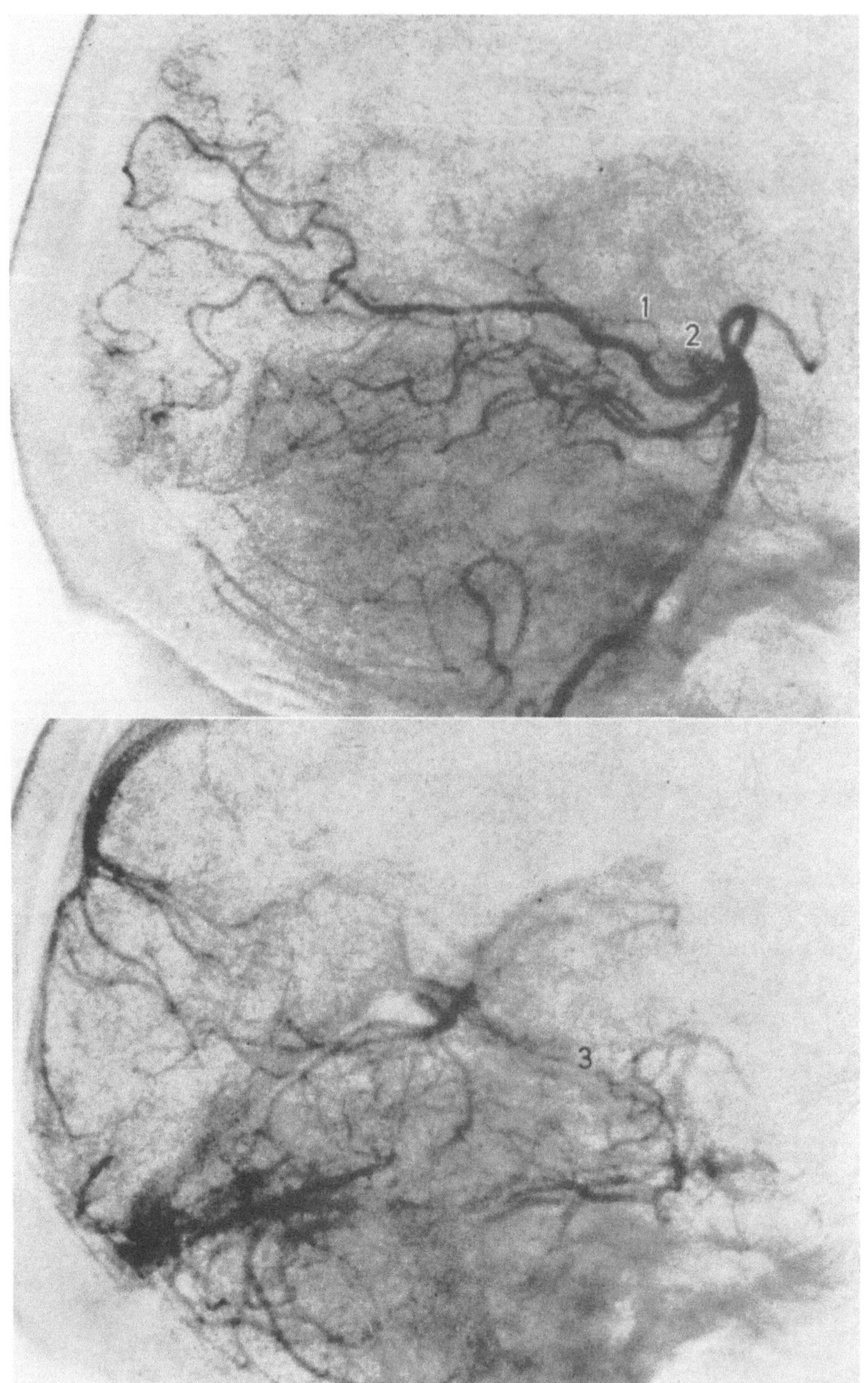

Fig. 88a

Fig. 88a and b. *Right thalamic tumour :* a) Hammock deformation of the posterior cerebral artery containing an overlying pathological arterial network. Blurred view of the basal vein: *1* Hammock. *2* Pathological network. *3* Blurred basal vein. b) Angiographic check-up I year later: *1* Displacement of the thalamo-perforating arteries to the left. These arteries are stretched and dilated. *2* Dilatation of the colliculi quadrigemini and corpori geniculati arteries. *3* and *4* Hypertrophy and deformations of the posterior choroidal arteries. *5* and *6* The mesencephalic venous system is blurred and faded

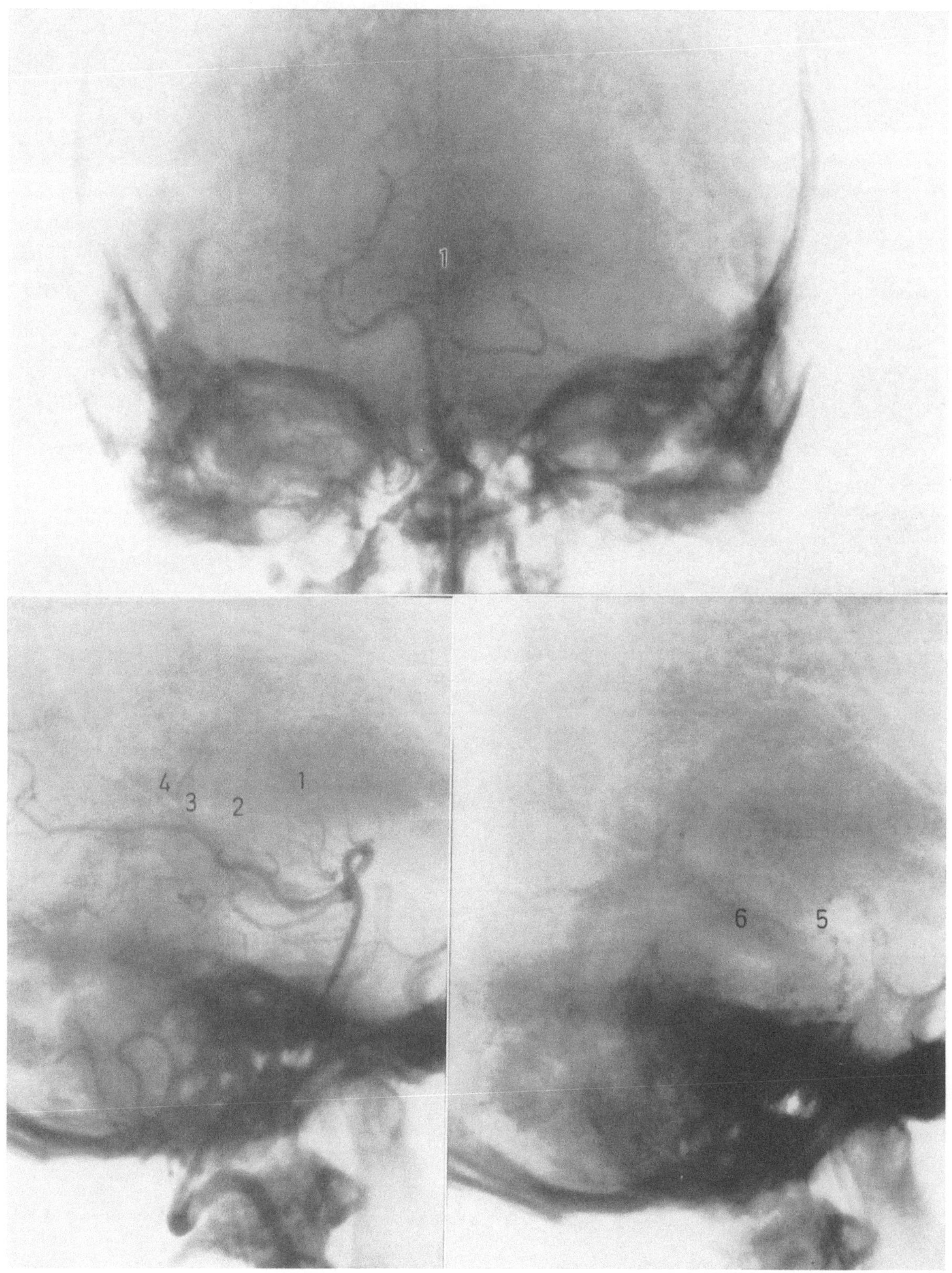

Fig. 88b

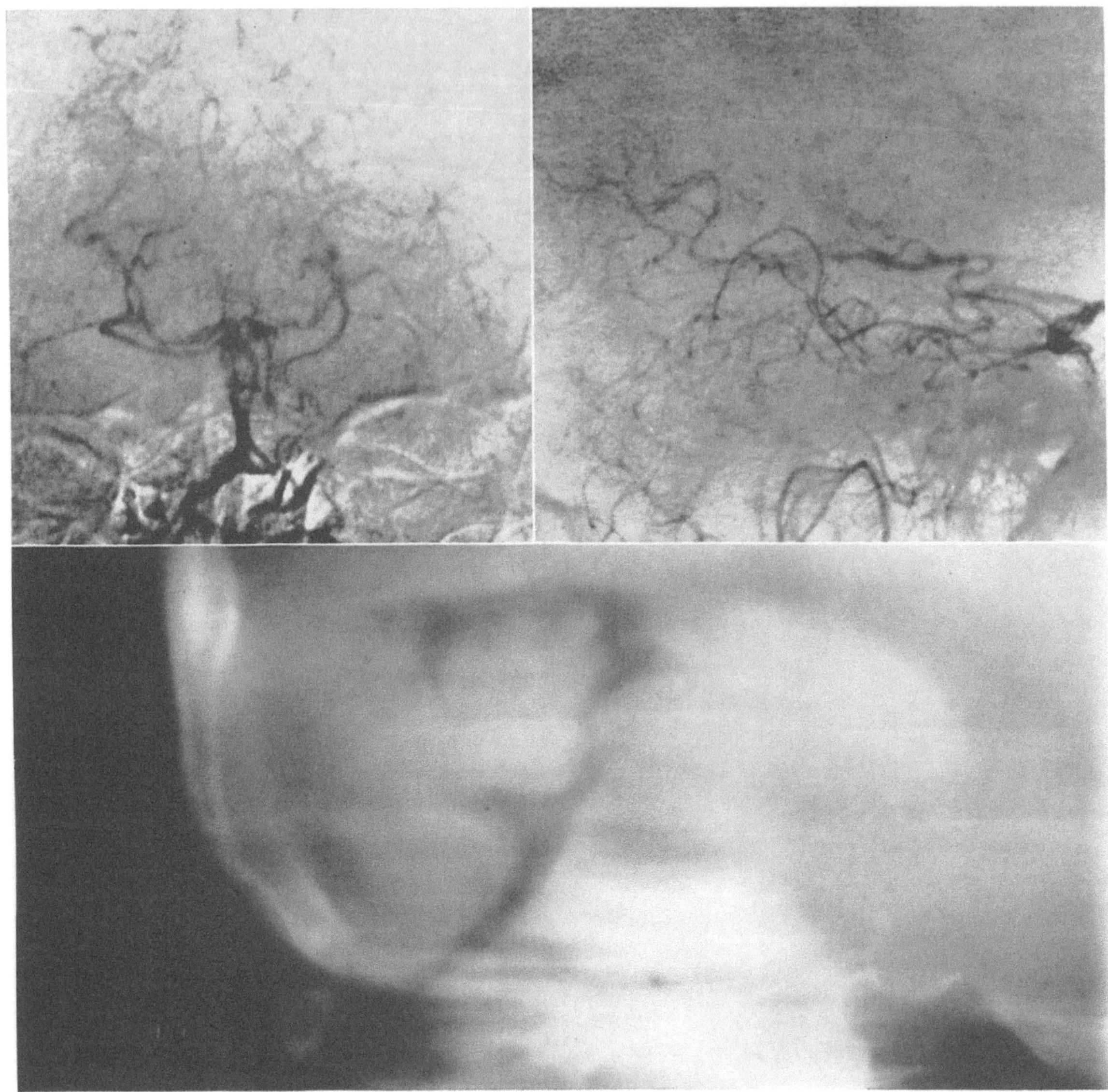

Fig. 89
Absence of the posterior choroidal arteries; dislocation and depression of the homolateral P2 segment
in the case of a thalamo-peduncular tumour

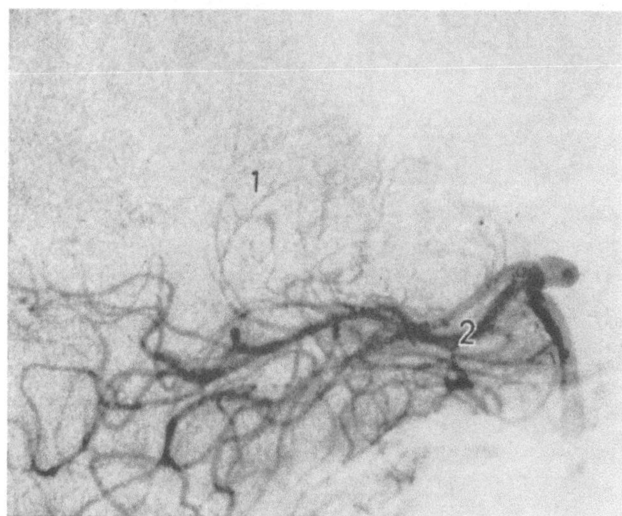

Fig. 90
Deep temporal tumour with encroachment of the posterior thalamus. *1* Increase of curvature in the postero-lateral choroidal arteries. *2* Homolateral depression of segment P2

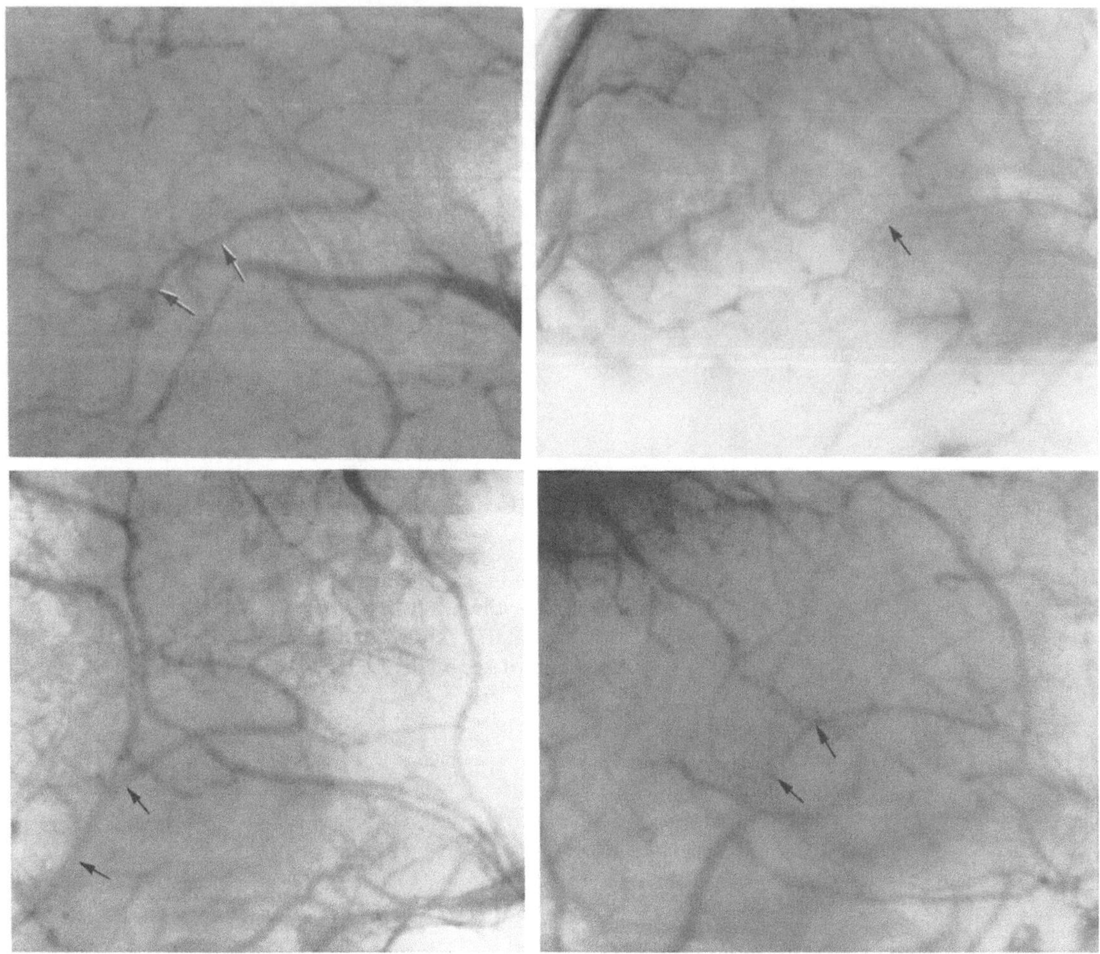

Fig. 91
Deformation and displacement of the internal cerebral vein in four cases of thalamic tumours, especially posterior

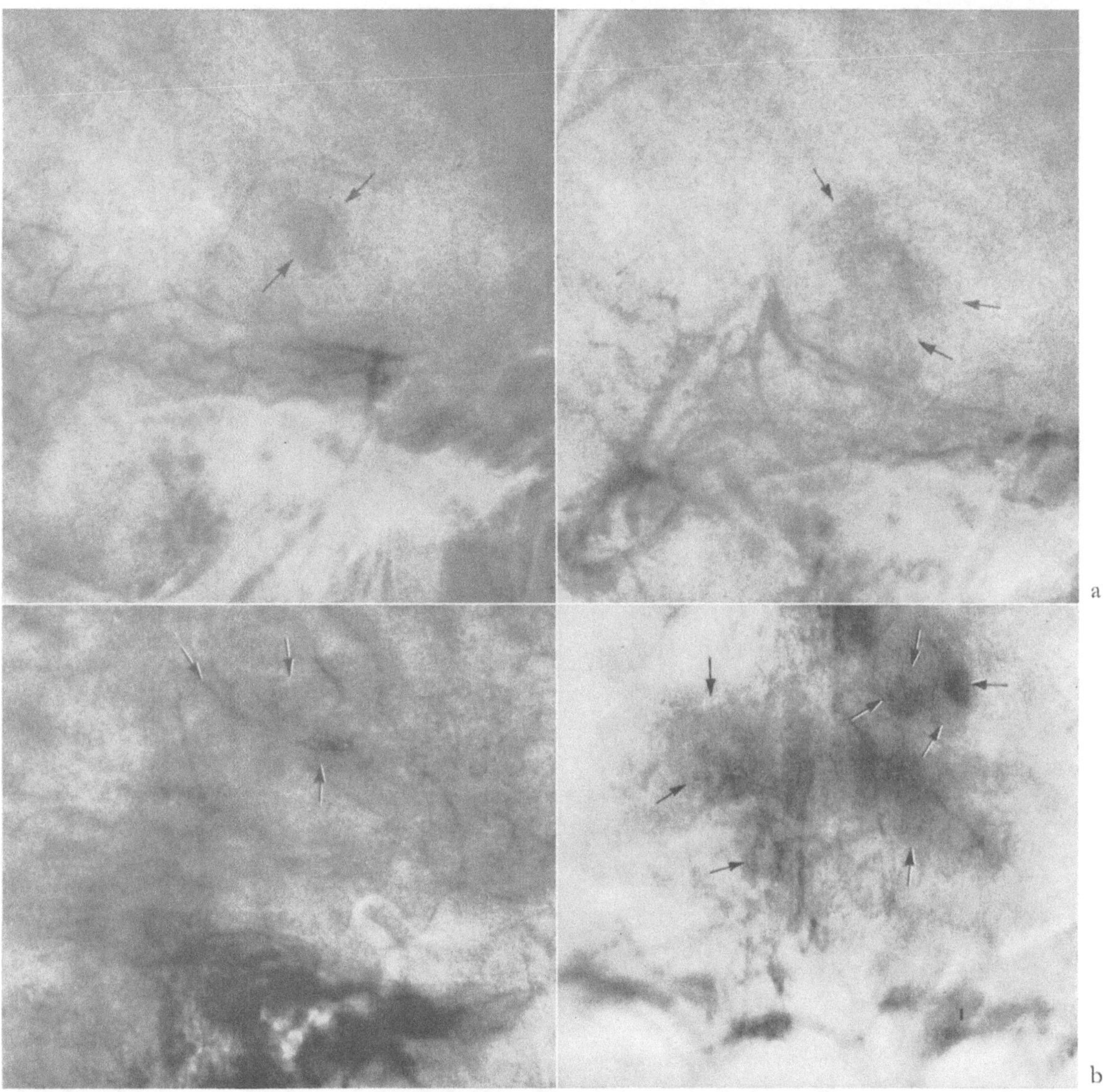

Fig. 92a and b
Thalamic capillarography in two cases of thalamic tumour. a) Small tumoral nucleus (lateral projection). b) Wide range of bilateral tumoral impregnation (lateral and frontal projection)

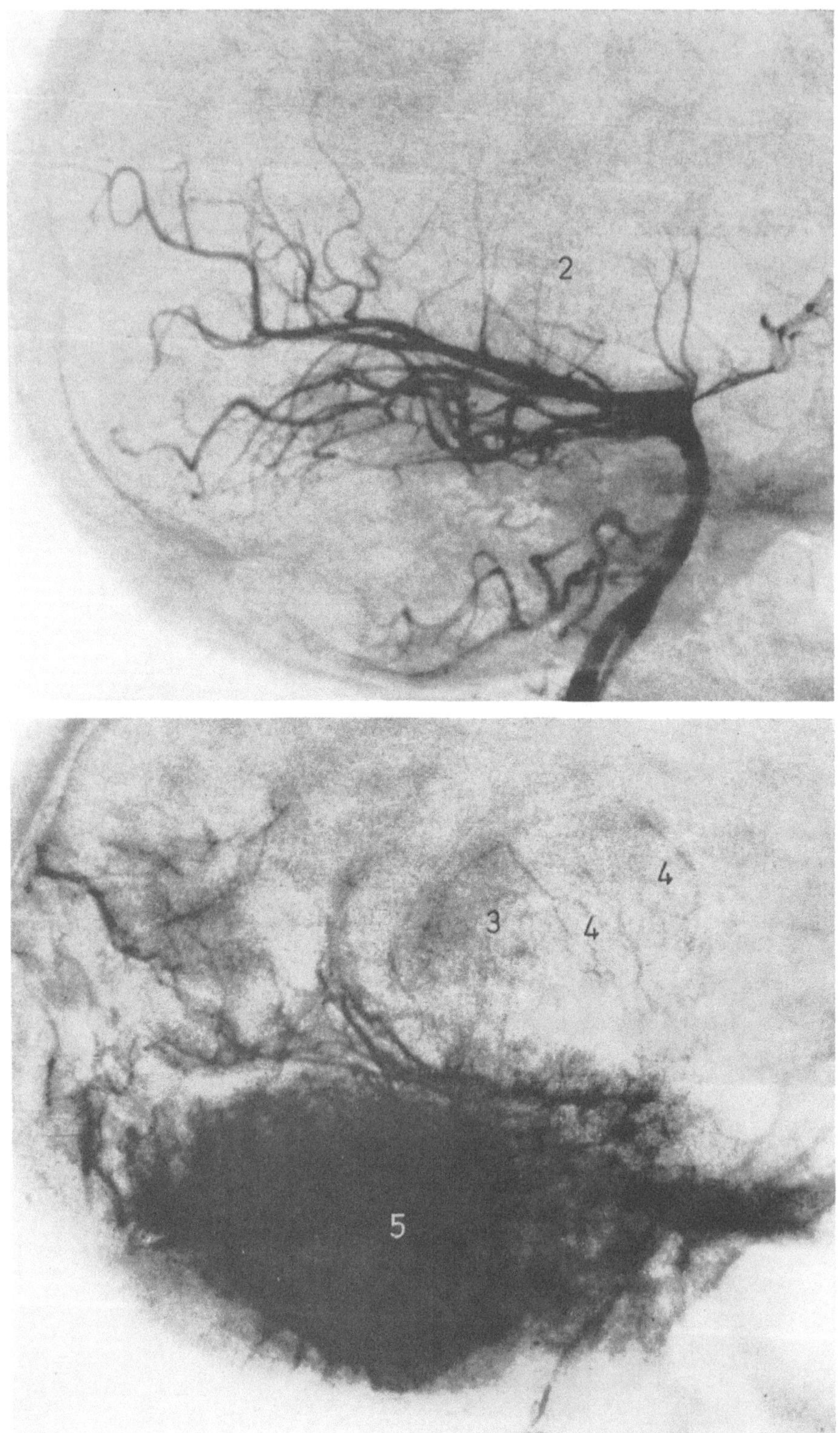

Fig. 93 a and b. Large thalamic tumour. *1* Dilated striothalamic vein. *2* Marked arterial deformation in the thalamo-mesencephalic region. *3* Tumoral capillarography. *4* Dilated thalamic vein. *5* Stasis in the posterior fossa

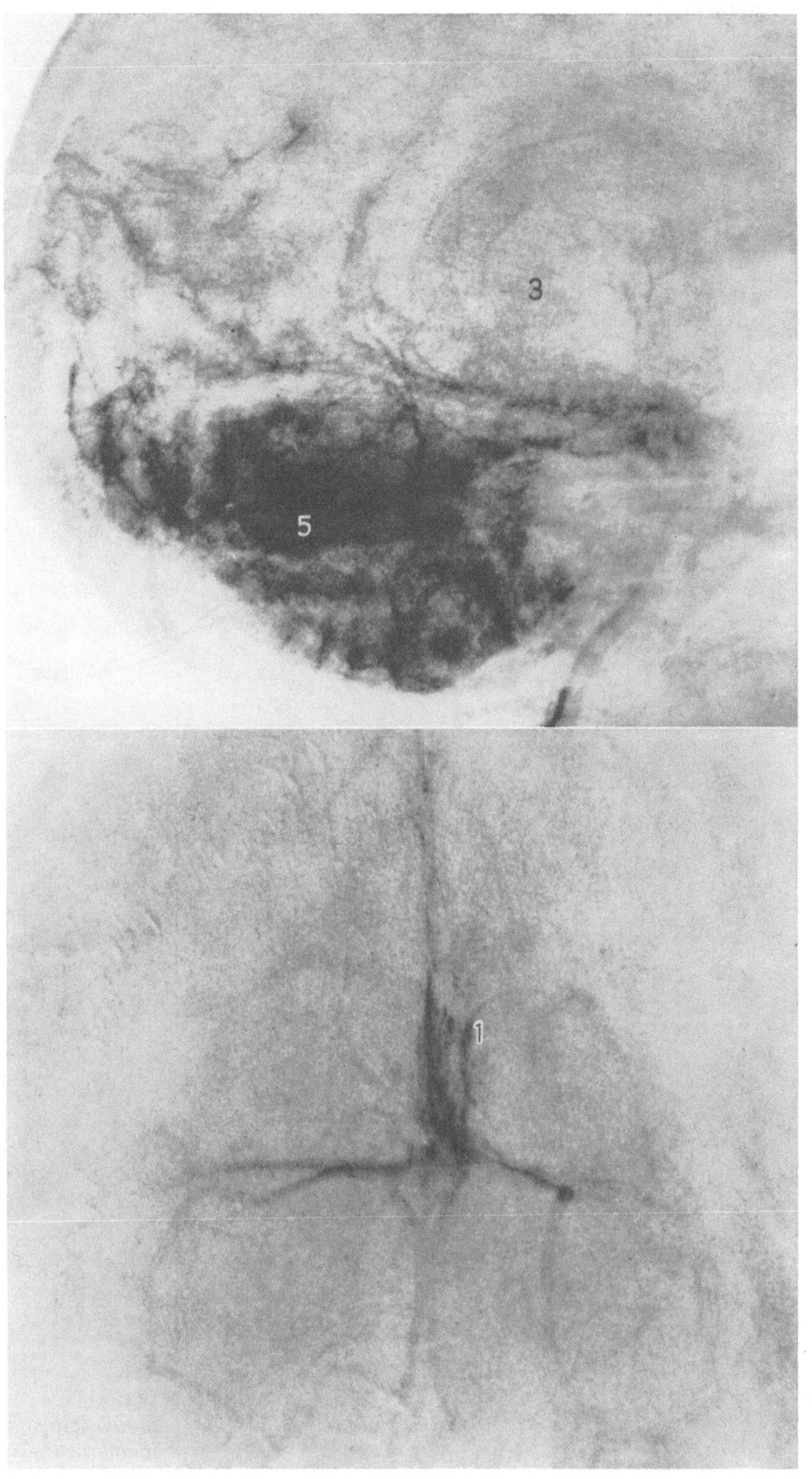

Fig. 93 b

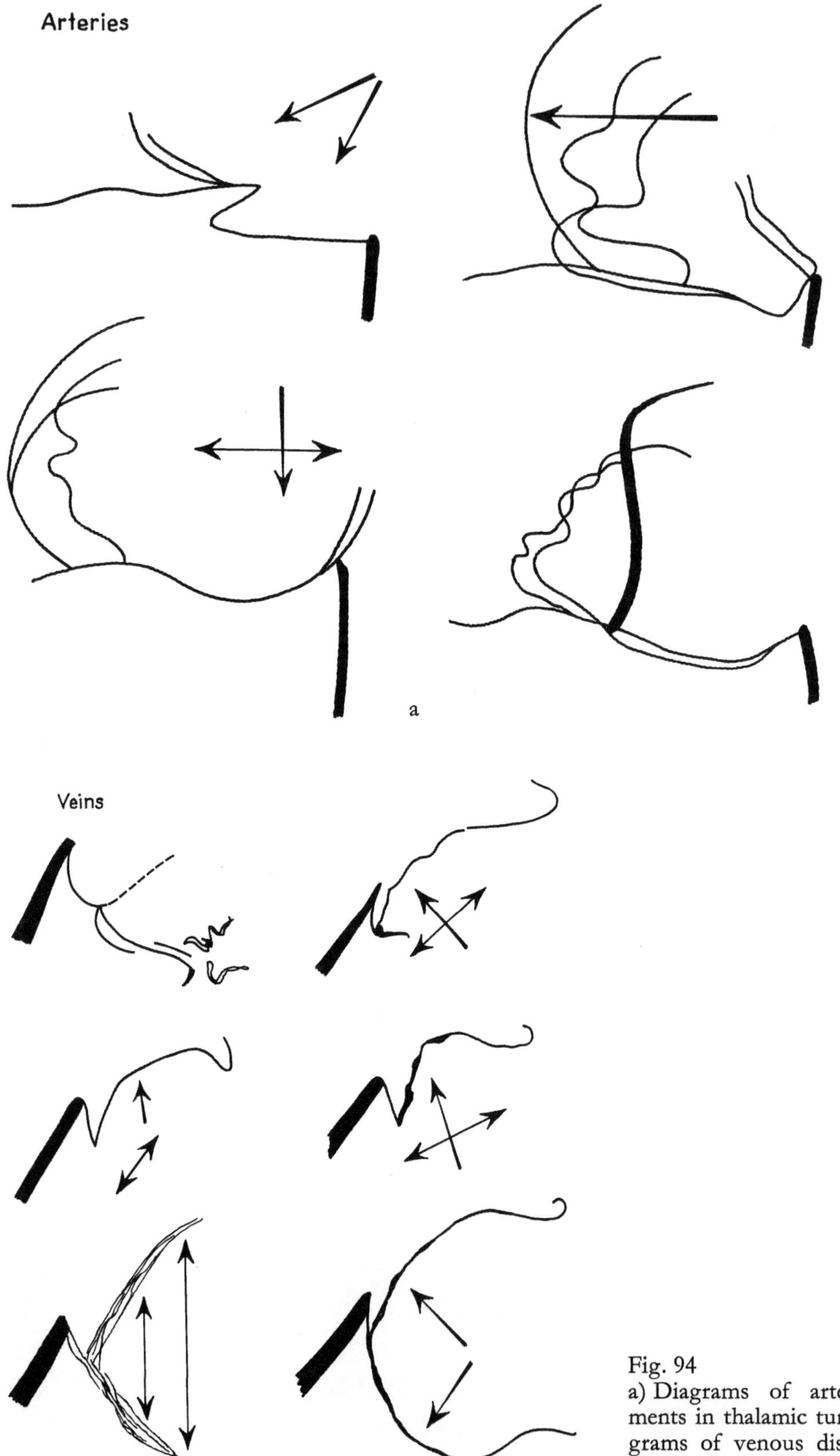

Fig. 94
a) Diagrams of arterial displacements in thalamic tumours. b) Diagrams of venous displacements in thalamic tumours

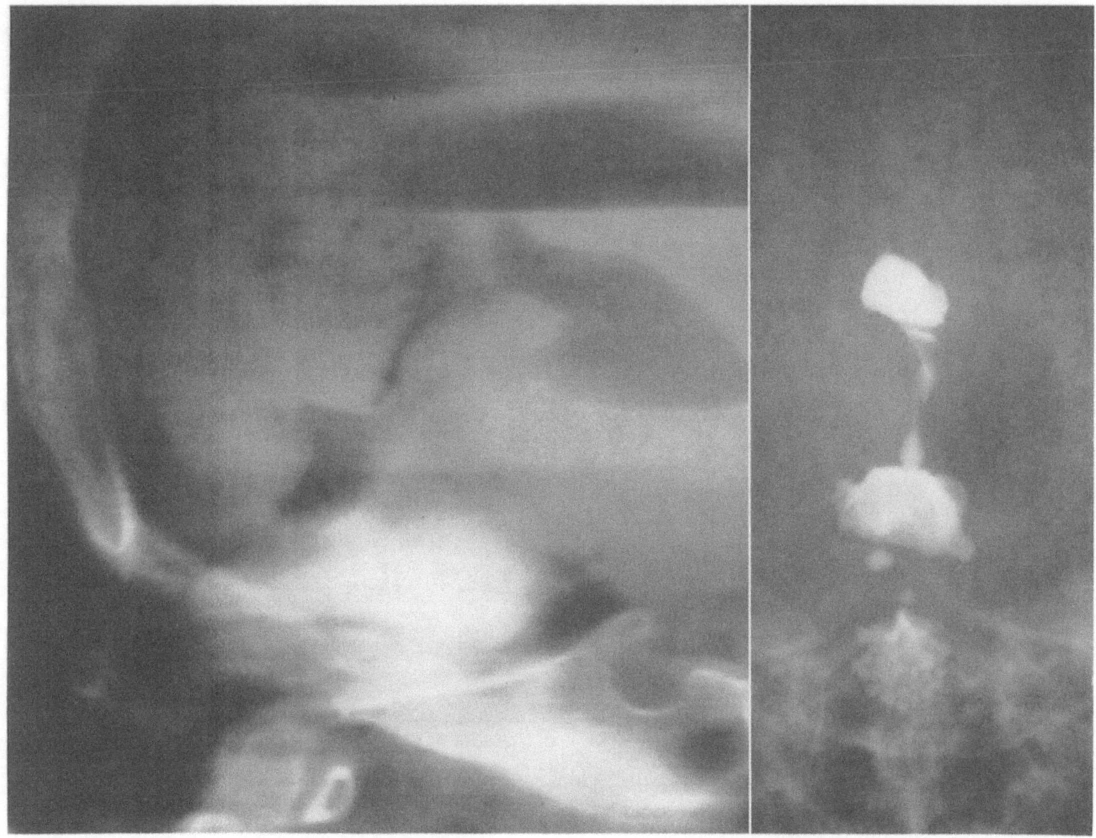

Fig. 95
Pneumoencephalography and pantopaque ventriculography in the case of a peduncular tumour

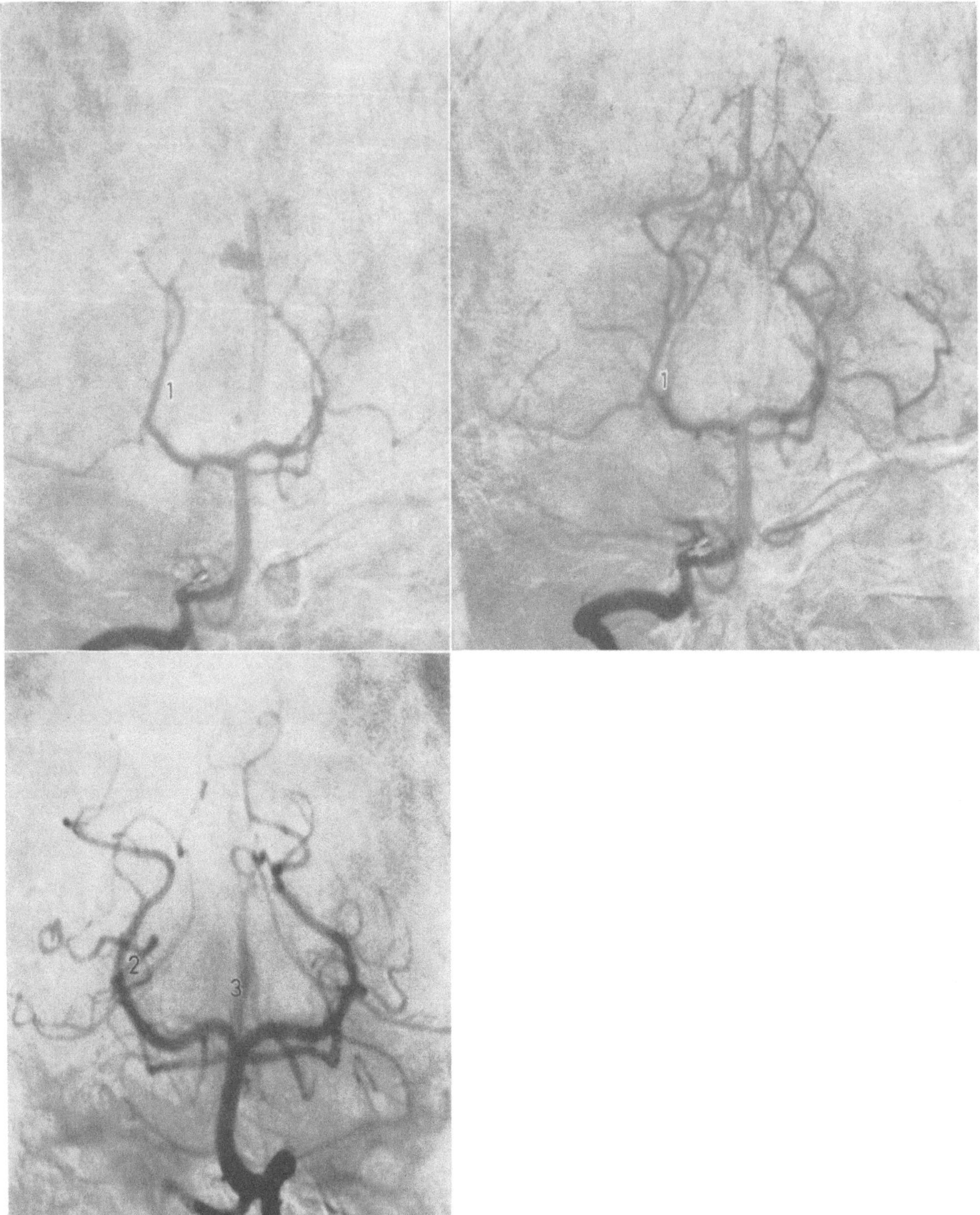

Fig. 96
Frontal arteriography of peduncular tumours. *1* Rigidity and angulation of the segments P1 and P2 (right peduncular tumour). *2* Increase in curvature of segment P1 and P2 (right peduncular tumour). *3* Deviation to the opposite side of the thalamo-perforating arteries (right peduncular tumour)

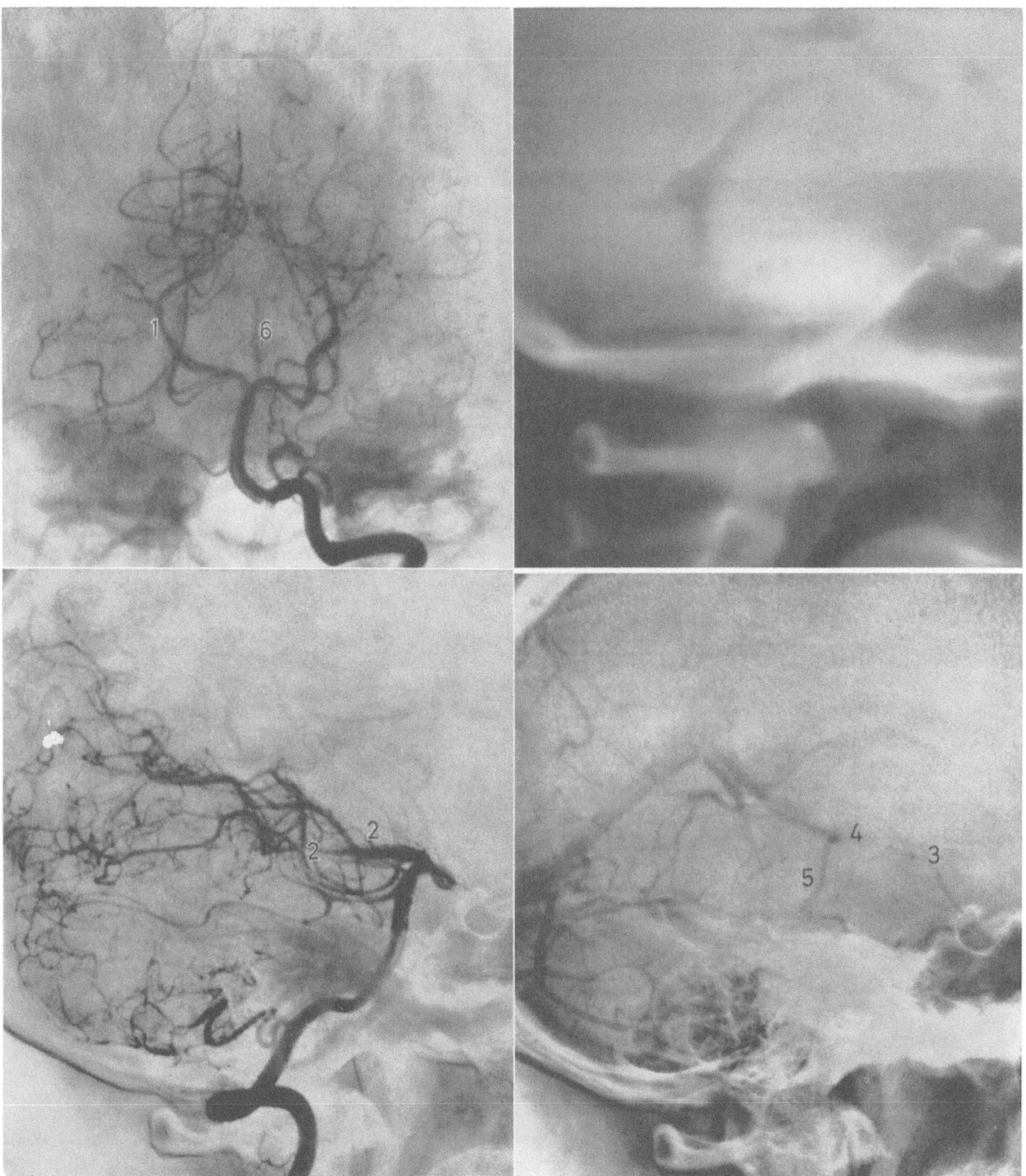

Fig. 97
Ponto-peduncular tumour. *1* Increase in curvature of the peripeduncular segments of the posterior cerebral artery on the tumour side. *2* Hammock of the latero-peduncular segment of the posterior cerebral artery and of the split postero-superior cerebellar artery. *3* Rigidity and elevation of the interpeduncular and prepontine veins. *4* Basal vein. *5* Dilatation of the lateral mesencephalic vein. *6* Deviation of the thalamo-perforating arteries towards the opposite side

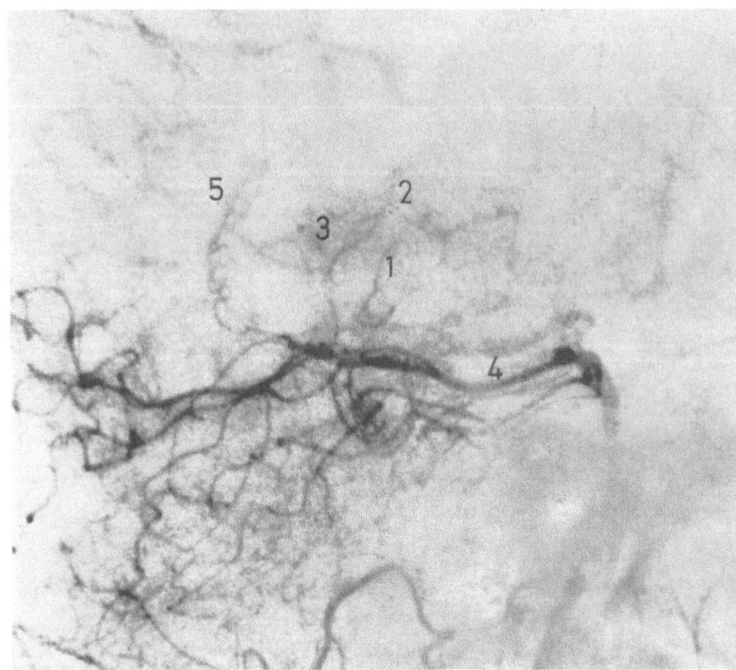

Fig. 98
Mesencephalic hematoma. Dislocation and deformation of the postero-medial (*1*) and lateral (*2*) choroidal arteries, tumoral capillarography (*3*), hammock of the latero-peduncular segment of the posterior cerebral artery (*4*), normal posterior pericallosal artery (*5*)

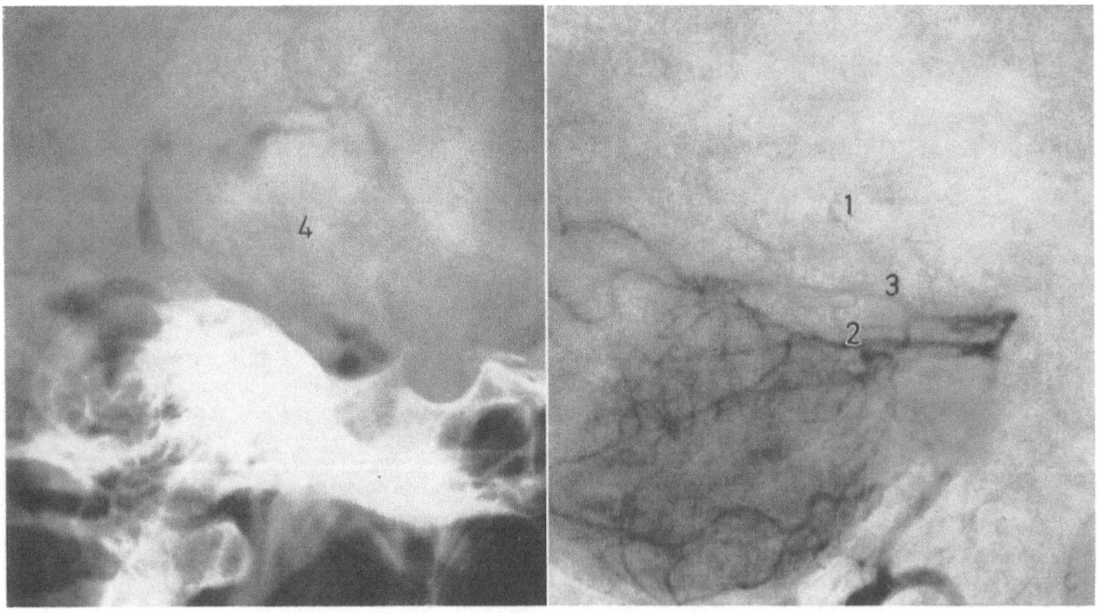

Fig. 99
Mesencephalic tumour. *1* Dislocation of the posterior choroidal arteries. *2* Hammock of the homolateral posterior cerebral artery. *3* Rigidity of the opposite posterior cerebral artery. *4* Pneumographic outline of the tumour

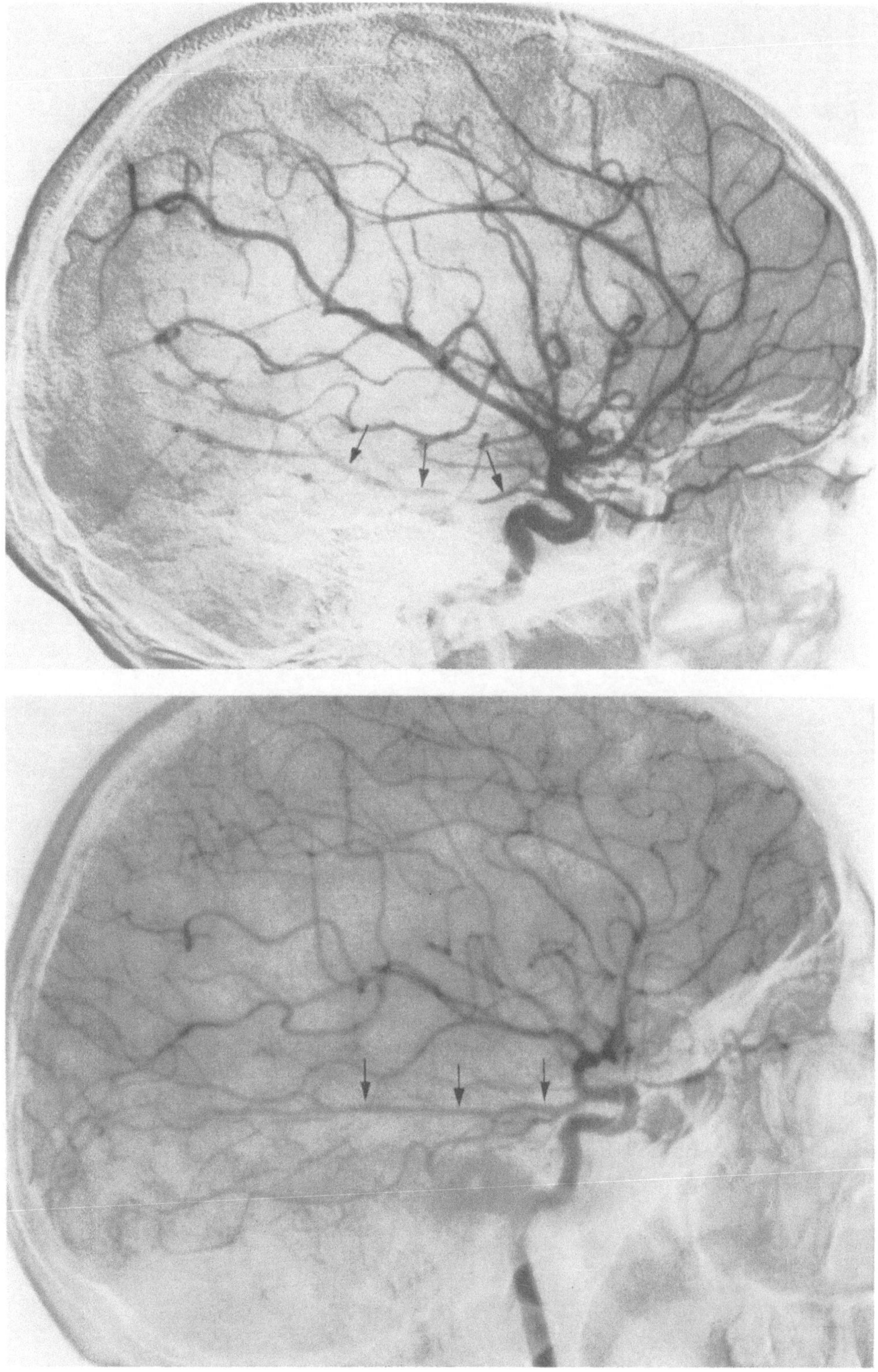

Fig. 100
Peduncular tumour : 2 cases. Carotid angiography: hammock sign of segment P2 above;
rigidity of P2 below

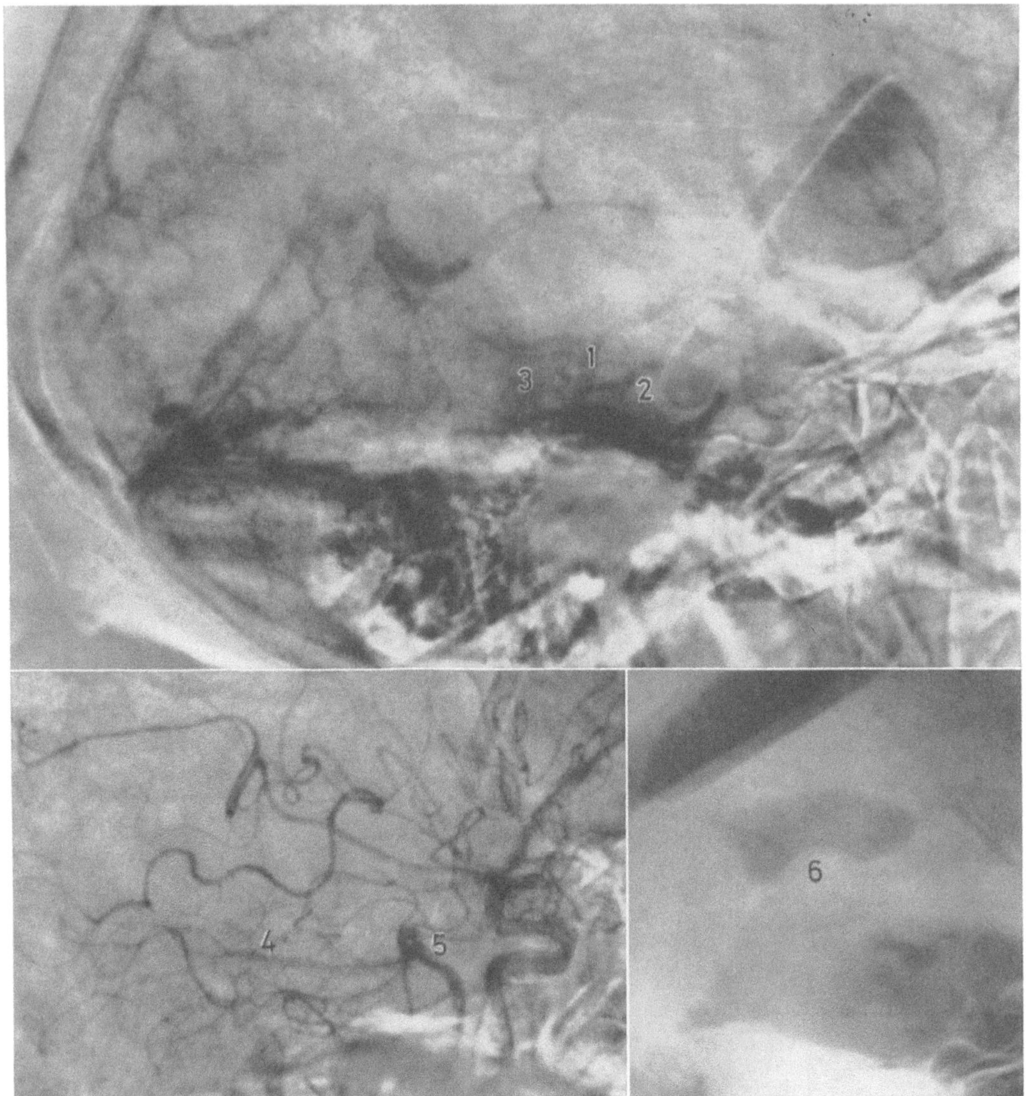

Fig. 101
Peduncular tumour. *1* Dislocation and dilatation of the terminal segment of the basal vein and of the lateral mesencephalic vein. *2* Dislocation and dilatation of the interpeduncular and prepontine venous system. *3* Tumoral capillarography. *4* Compression of segment P2. *5* Angulation of the superior extremity of the basilar trunk by the tumour. *6* Tumoral trace on the floor of the IIIrd ventricle

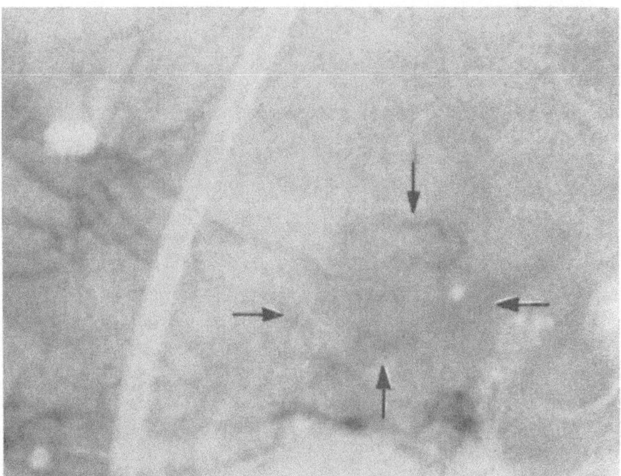

Fig. 102
Capillarography of a peduncular tumour

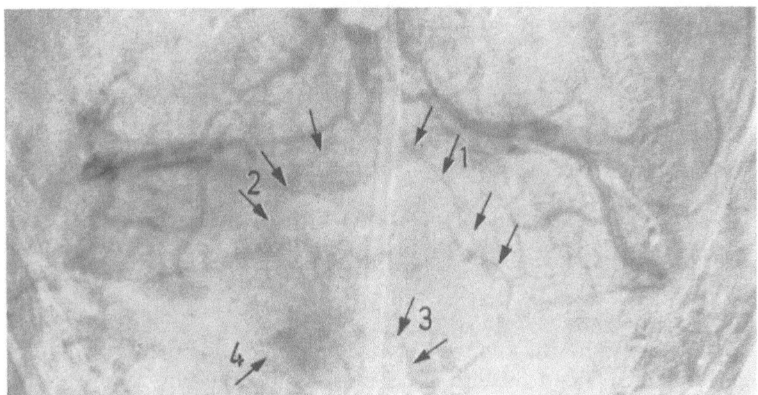

Fig. 103
Right peduncular tumour: vertebral phlebography. *1* Normal postero-lateral mesencephalic vein.
2 Posterior mesencephalic vein, thready above and absent below. *3* Normal interpeduncular vein.
4 Absence of the interpeduncular vein and tumoral capillarography

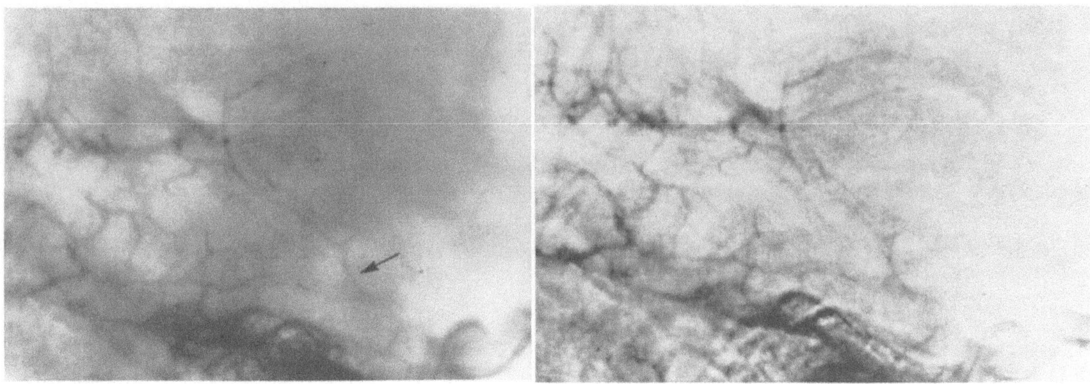

Fig. 104
Peduncular tumour seen as a trace on the peduncular vein

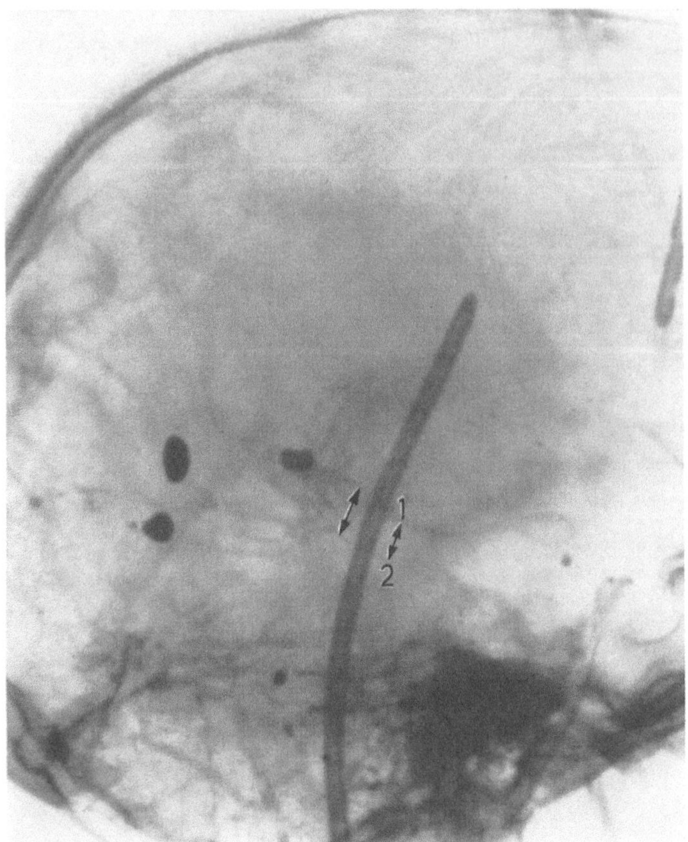

Fig. 105
Peduncular tumour. Venous dissociation in lateral projection
of the basal (*1*) and posterior mesencephalic (*2*) veins

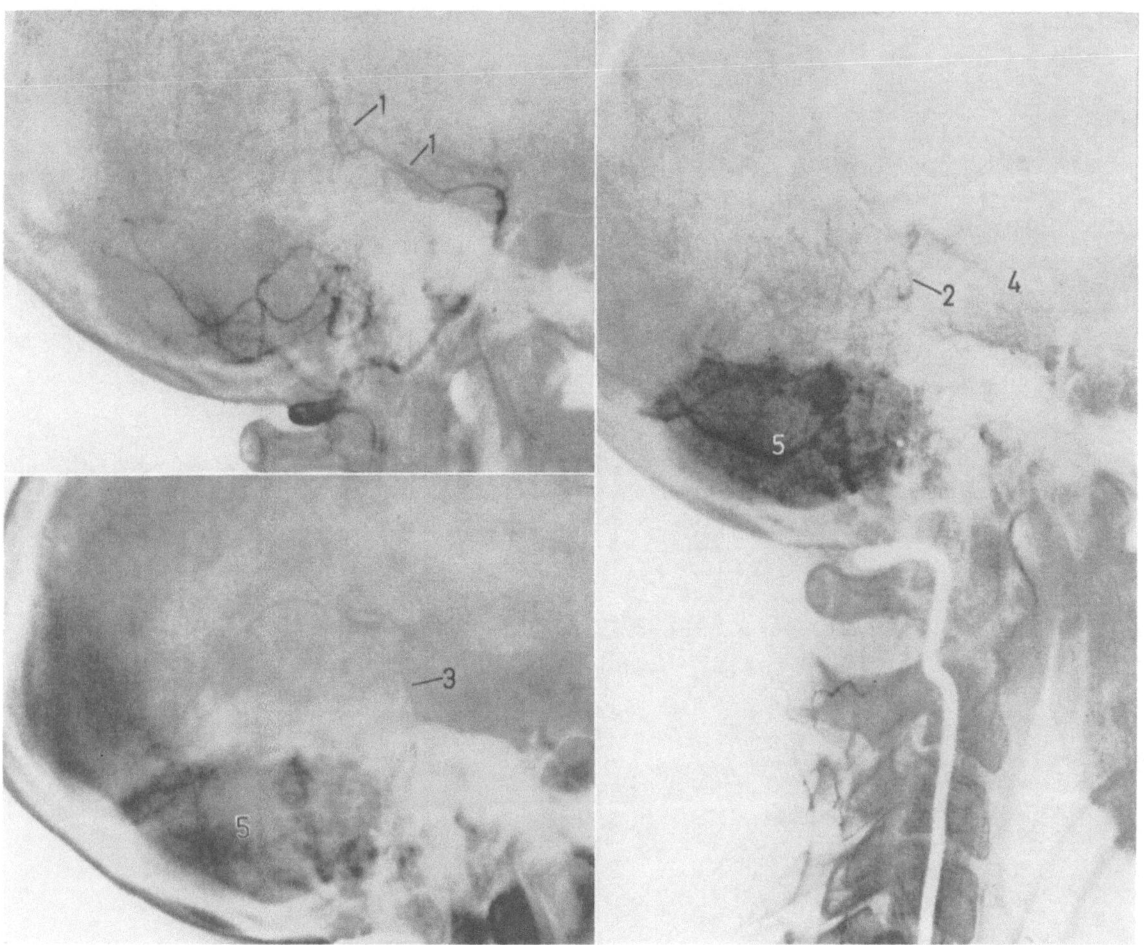

Fig. 106
Craniopharyngioma with a posterior development. *1* Hammock of segment P2. *2* Deformation and displacement of the precentral vein. *3* Deformation and displacement of the lateral mesencephalic vein. *4* Dislocation of the interpeduncular veins. *5* Capillarography of the posterior fossa (intracranial hypertension)

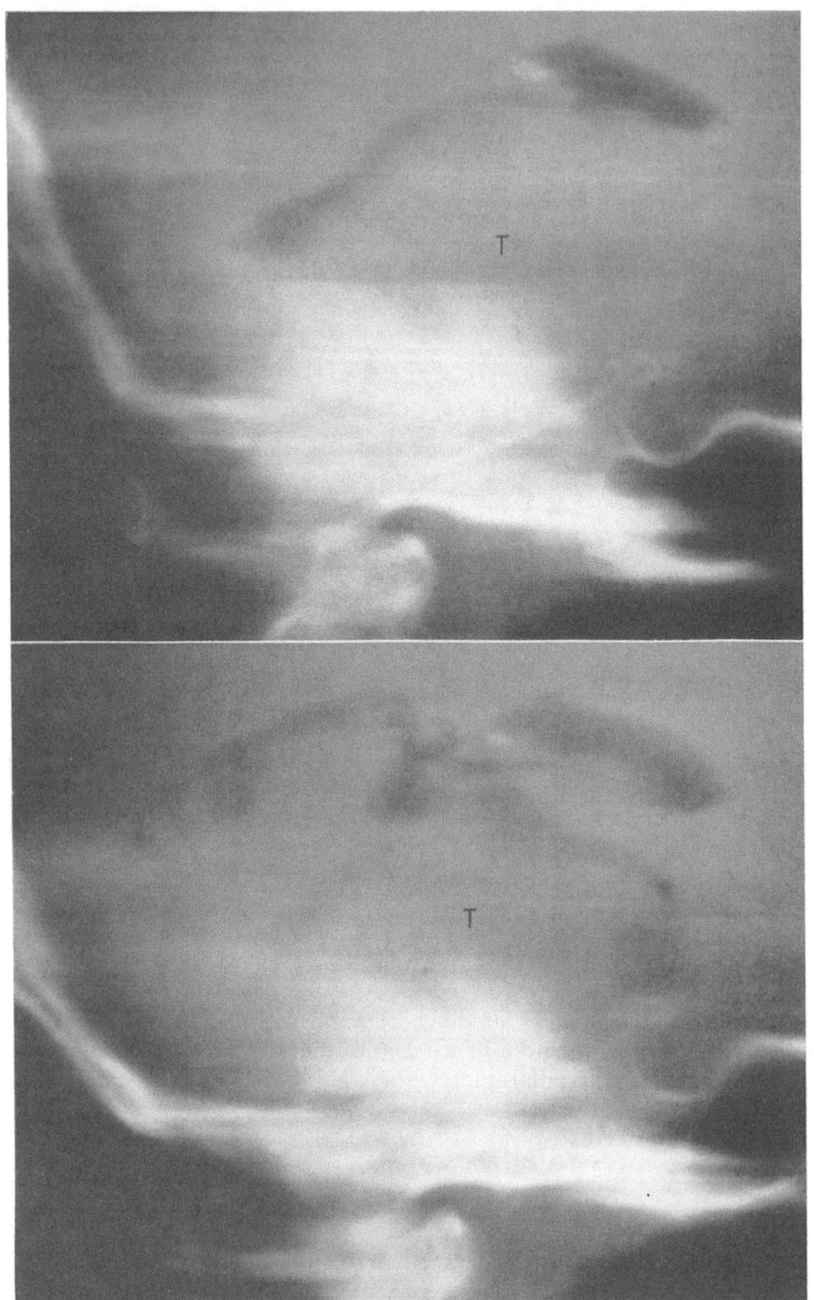

Fig. 107a

Fig. 107a and b
Extra-cerebral mass in the ponto-cerebellar angle. a) Pneumography.
b) Angiography. *1* Elevation of the peduncular vein. *2* Dilatation of the
lateral mesencephalic vein. *3* Increase in curvature of the prepontine vein.
4 Dissociation between the posterior mesencephalic vein and the basal
vein. *5* Important displacements of segments P1 and P2

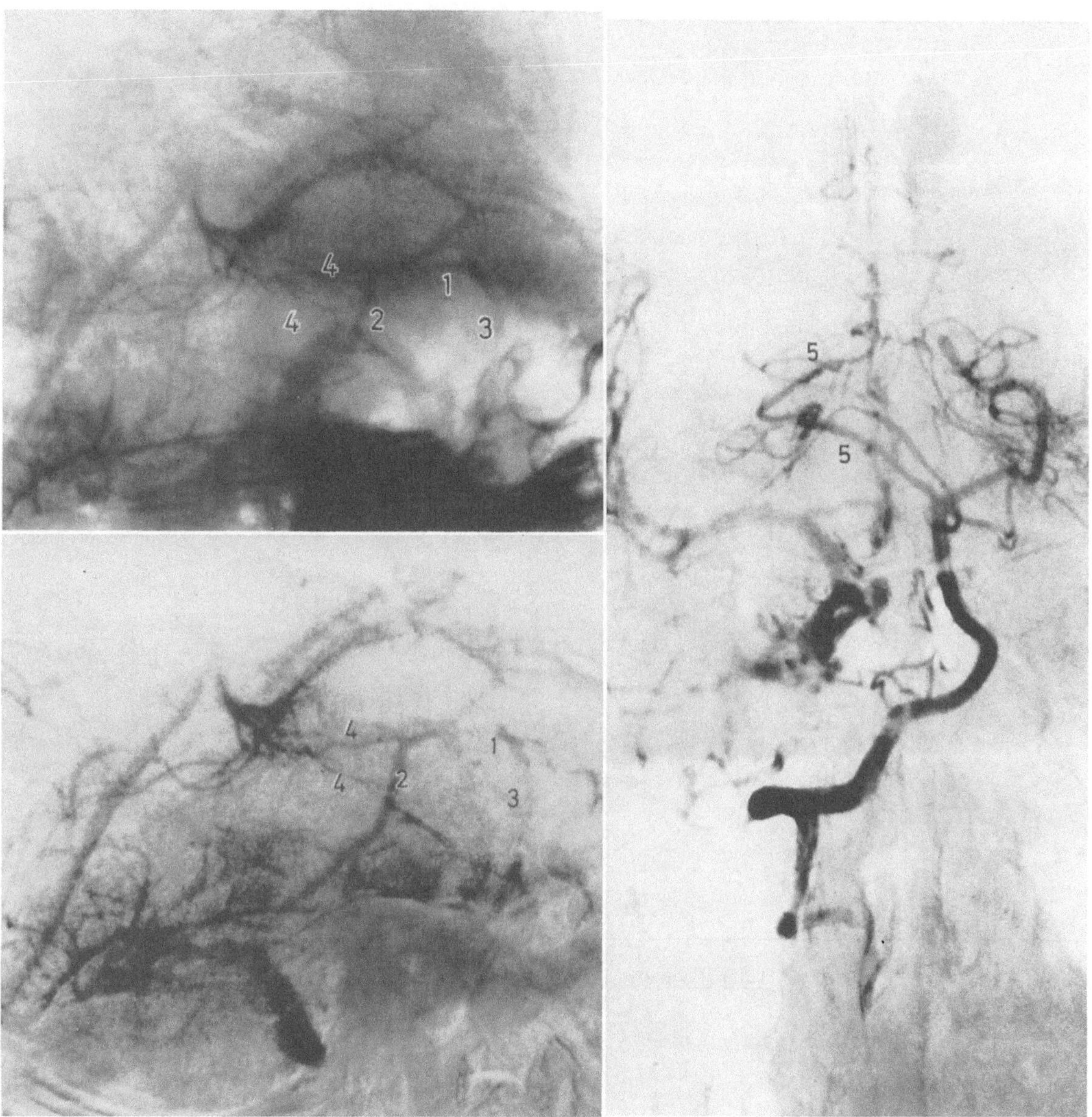

Fig. 107 b

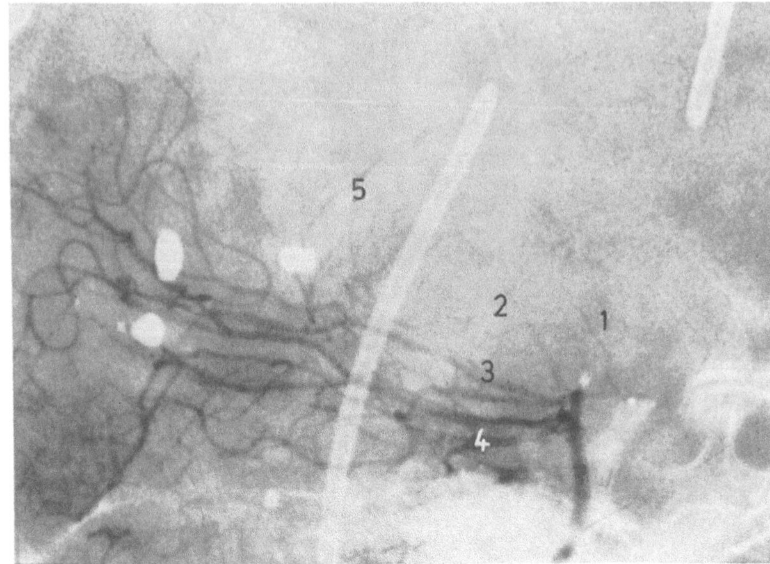

Fig. 108
Peduncular tumour with thalamic expansion.
1 Stretching of the anterior thalamo-perforating arteries. *2* Stretching of the posterior thalamo-perforating arteries.
3 Rigidity of P2.
4 Hammock of P2.
5 Increase in curvature of the posterior choroidal arteries

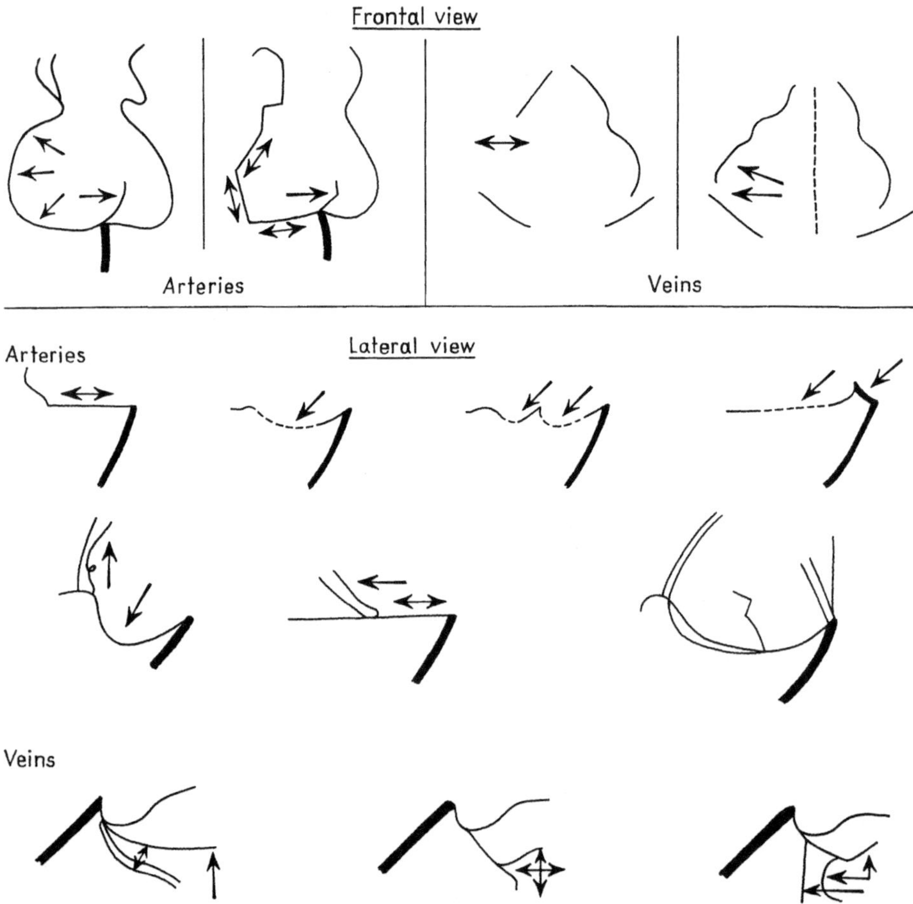

Fig. 109
Diagrams of arterial and venous deformations of peduncular tumours

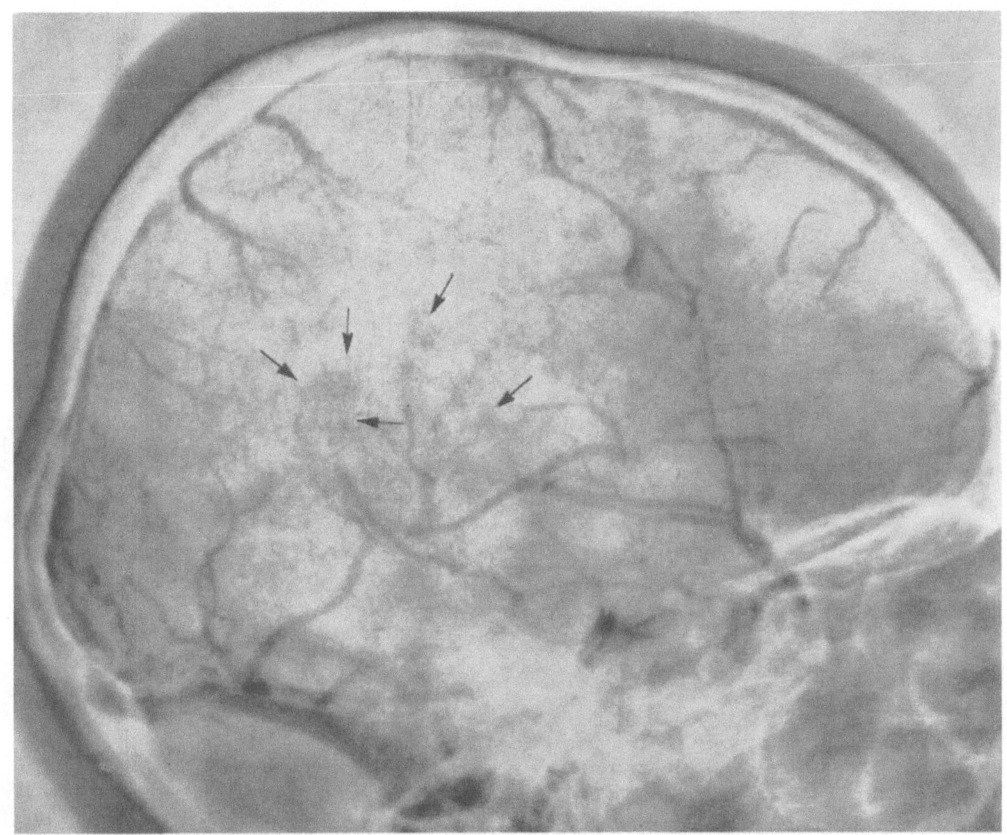

Fig. 110
Capillarography of a tumour of the splenium corporis callosi

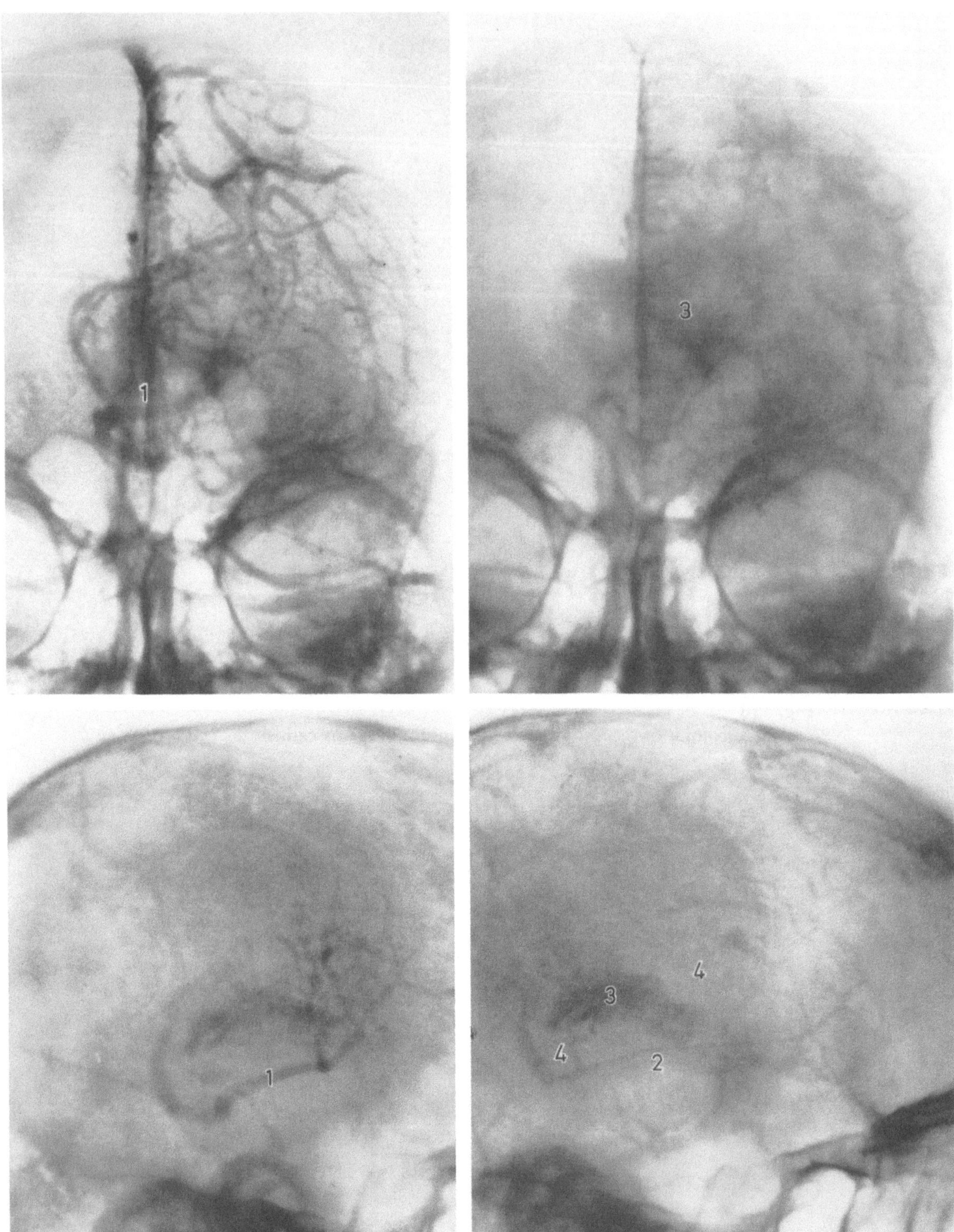

Fig. 111
Lateral intraventricular ependymoma invading the IIIrd ventricle. *1* Dilatation of the deep venous system. *2* Rigidity and angulation of the internal cerebral vein. *3* Tumoral capillarography of the venous phase. *4* Dilated ventricular veins

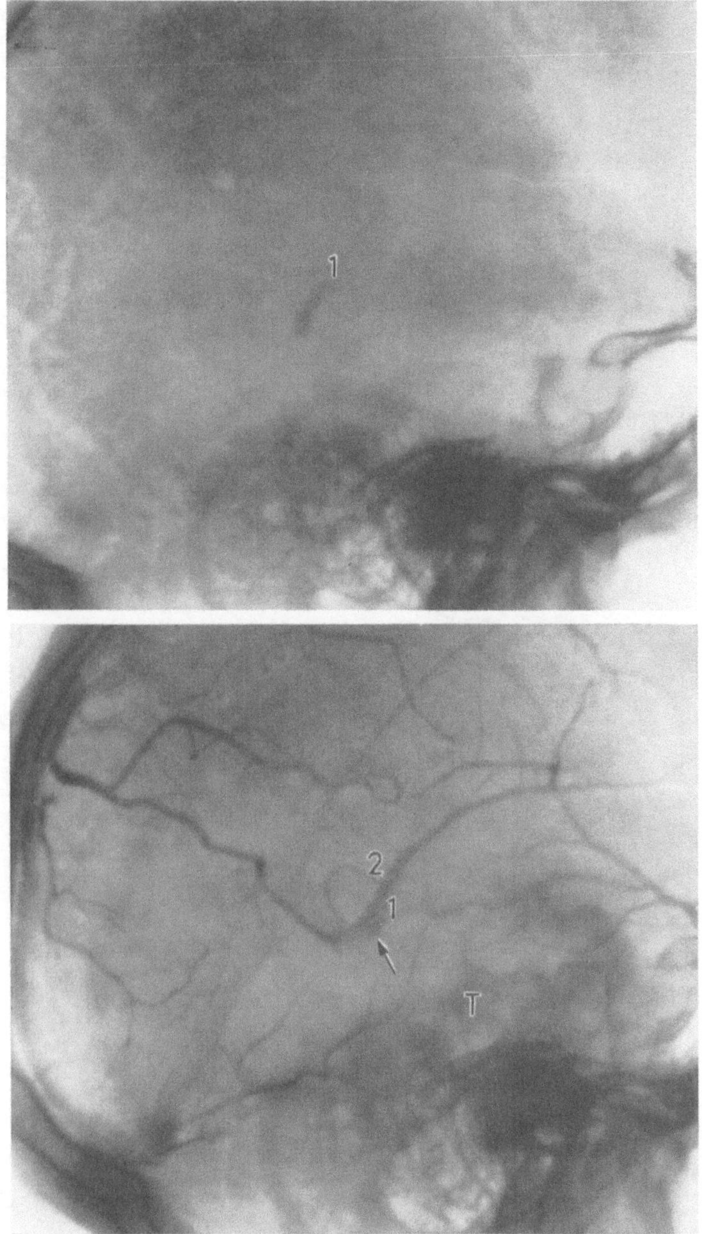

Fig. 112
Meningioma of the tentorium. Elevation of the calcified pineal gland (*1*) bringing it in contact with the internal cerebral vein (*2*). Compare with Fig. 73

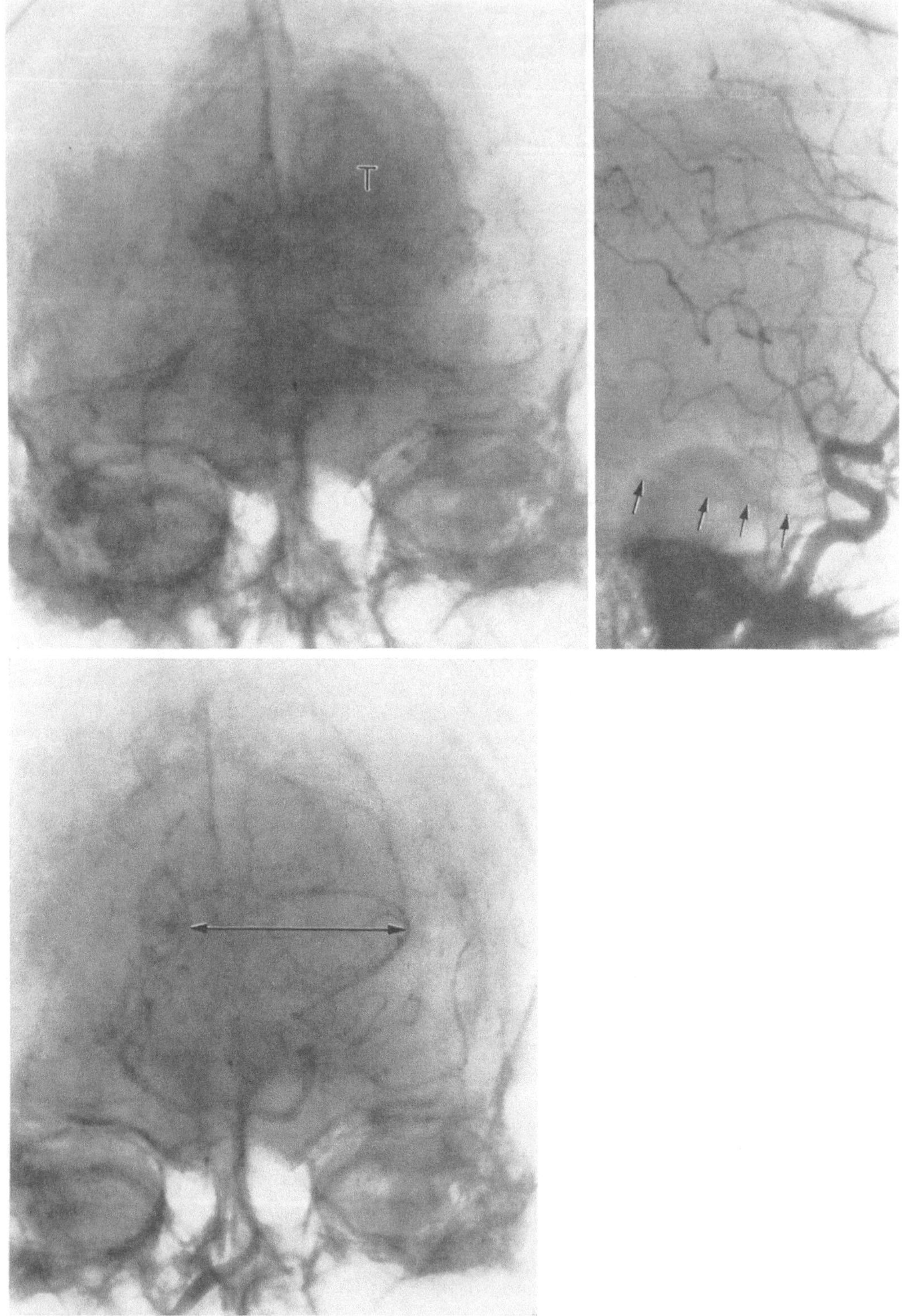

Fig. 113
Meningioma of the tentorium. Strong displacement of the posterior cerebral arteries. Tumoral capillarography. Tentorial arteries of the internal carotid

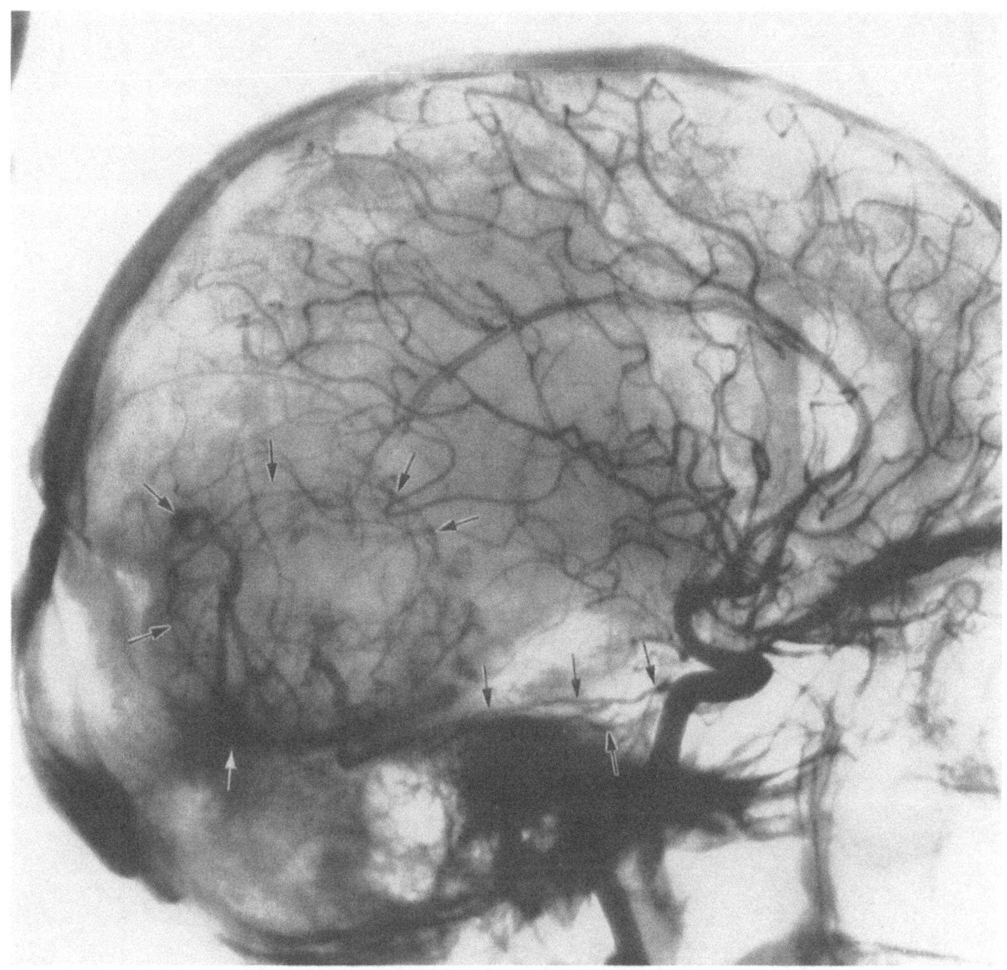

Fig. 114
Meningioma of the tentorium with numerous bordering vessels and hypertrophy of the
tentorial branches of the internal carotid

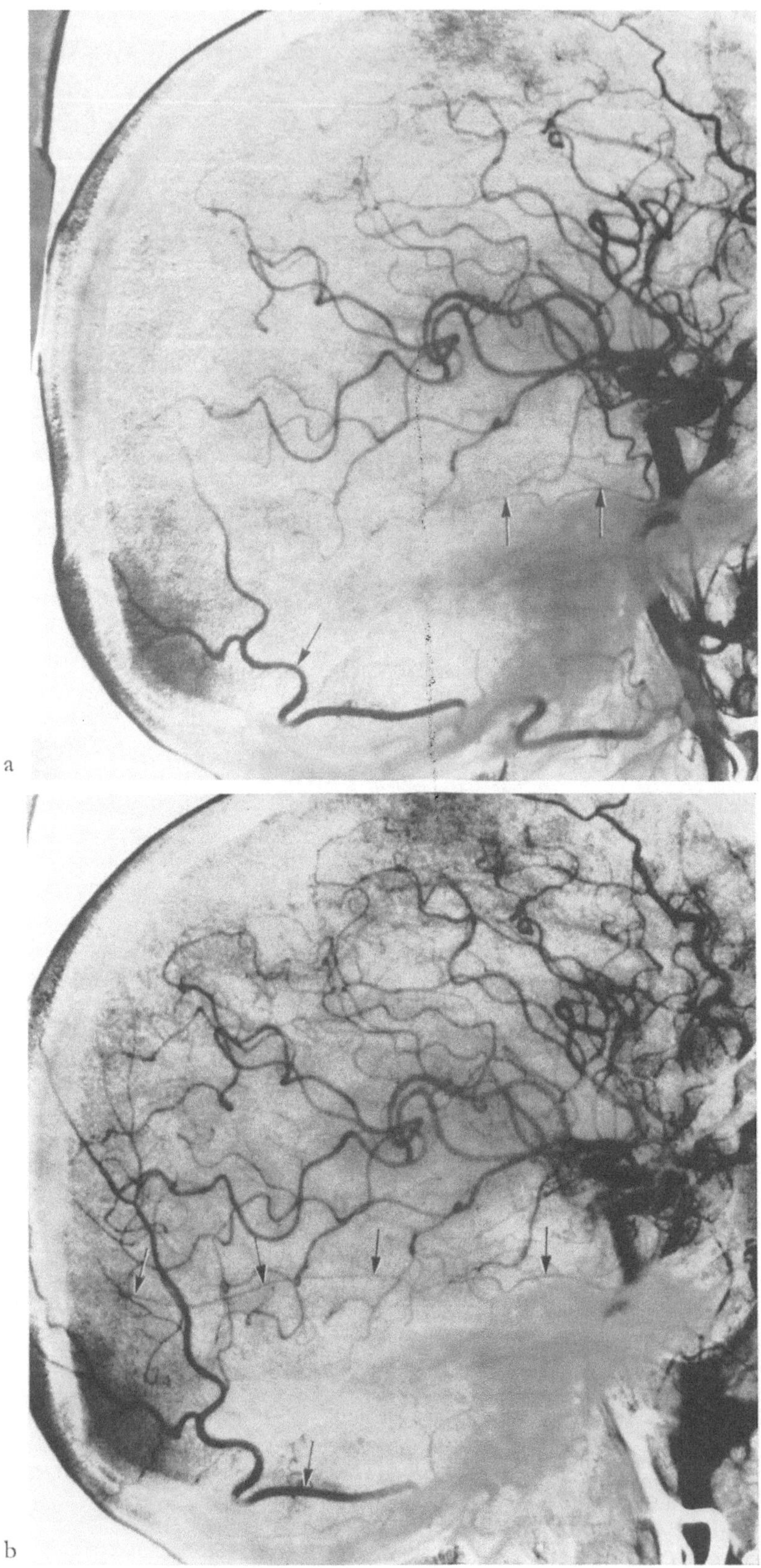

Fig. 115a–d. Meningioma of the tentorium. Hypertrophy of the tentorial branches of the carotid artery and of the occipital artery

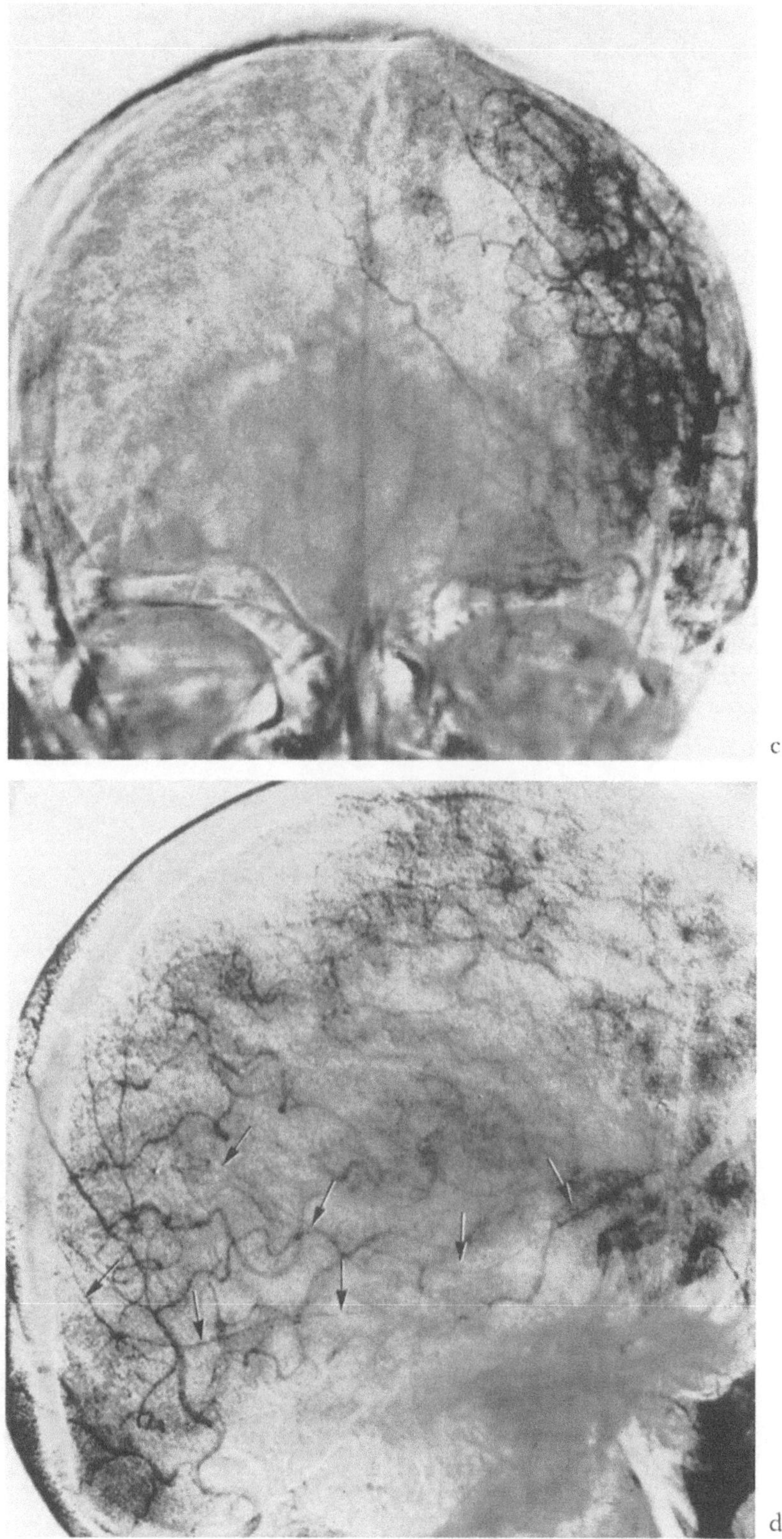

Fig. 115c and d

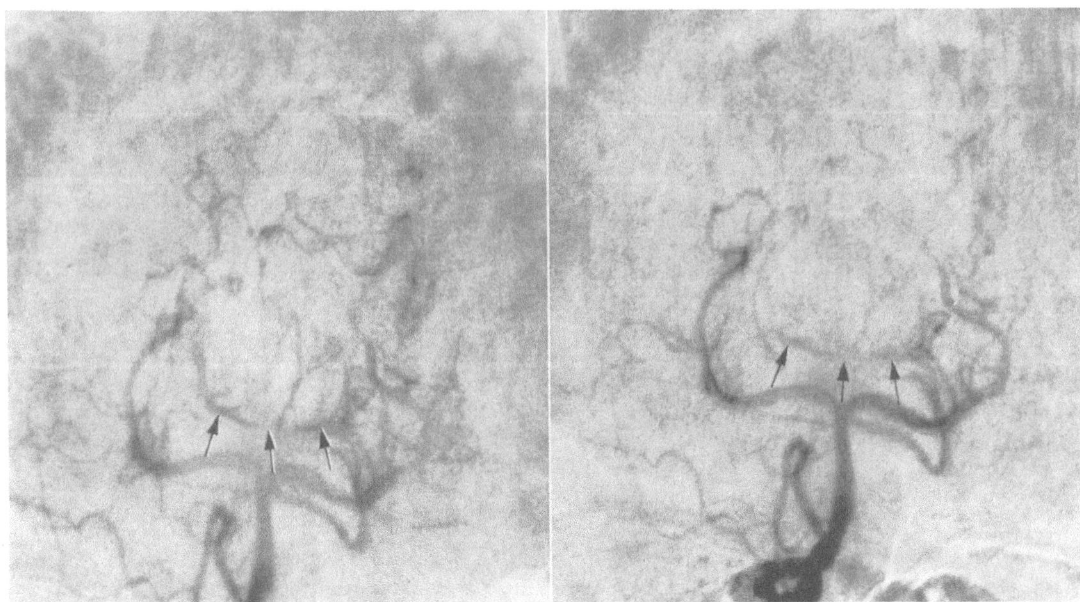

Fig. 116
Meningioma of the tentorium. Arterial "hammock" shape delimiting the inferior pole of the tumour. Compare this image with figures 25 and 81 (pineal artery and "hammock" in pinealomas). Contrary to the pinealoma, the meningioma displaces the posterior cerebral arteries

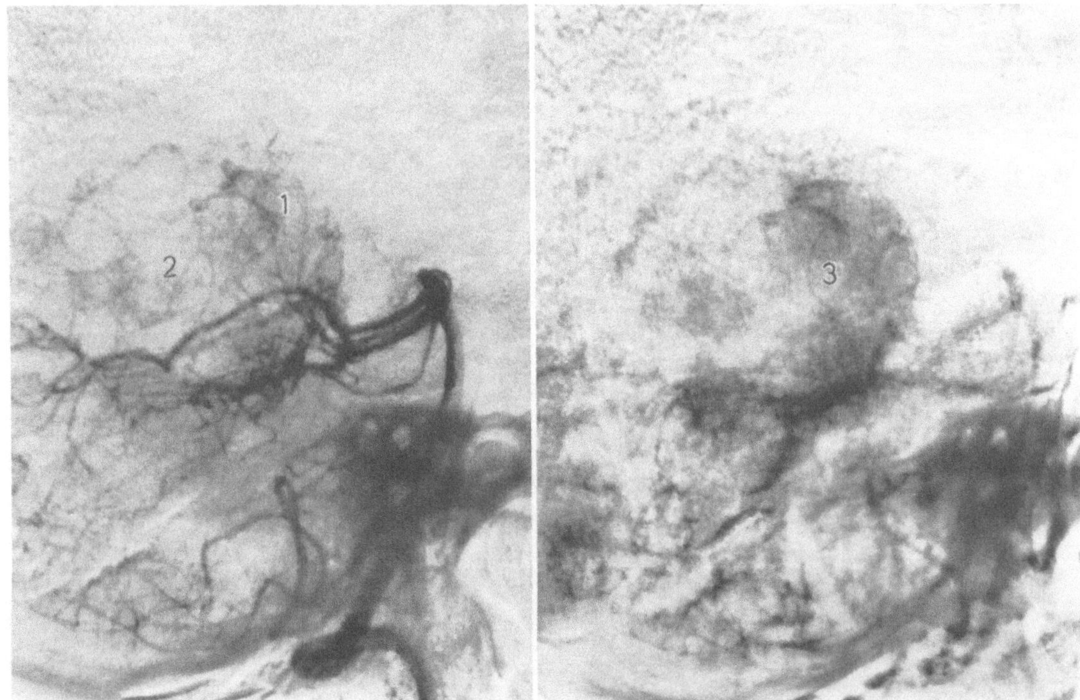

Fig. 117
Meningioma of the tentorium. *1* Dislocation of the posterior choroidal arteries embodied in the tumour. *2* Sharp angulation of the posterior pericallosal artery. *3* Tumoral capillarography

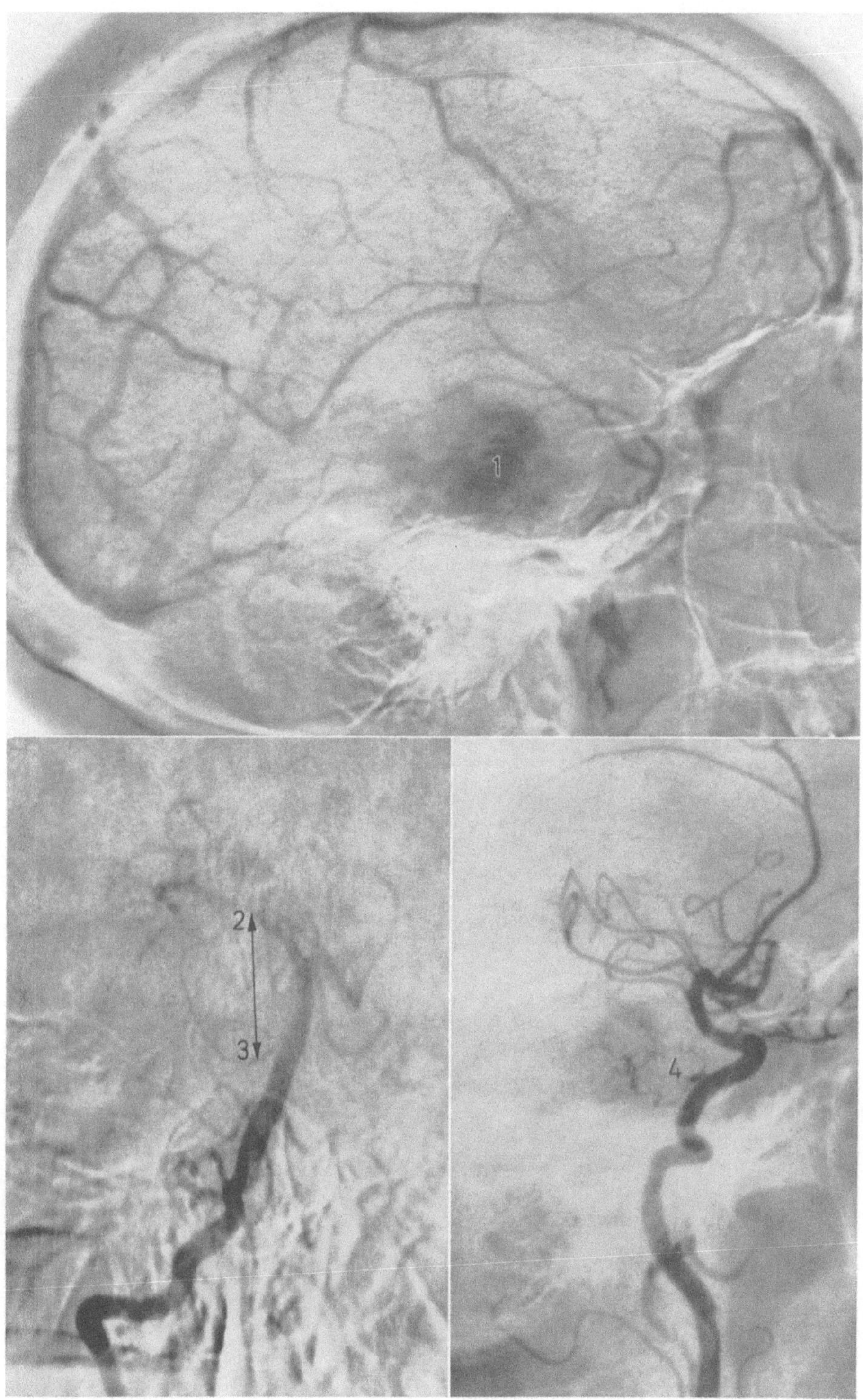

Fig. 118
Dissociation of the posterior cerebral artery (*2*) and the superior cerebellar artery (*3*)
due to the expansion of a tentorial meningioma. Tumoral capillarography (*1*).
Tentorial branches of the internal carotid (*4*)

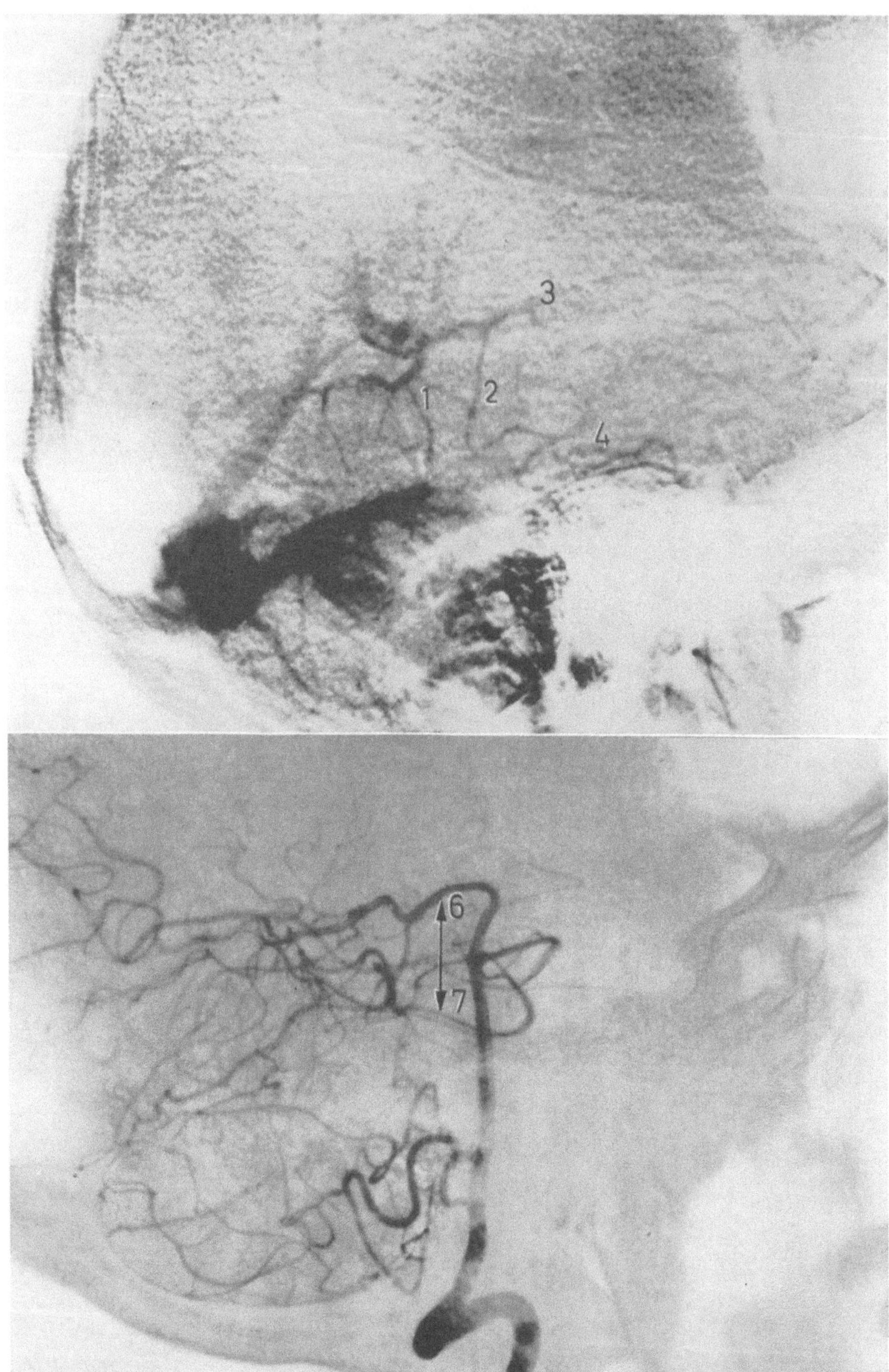

Fig. 119 a
Dissociation of the posterior cerebral artery (*6*) and the postero-superior cerebellar artery (*7*) due to expansion of a meningioma in the tentorium (*T*): *1* Backward displaced precentral vein. *2* Displaced lateral mesencephalic vein. *3* Elevated basal vein. *4* Compressed prepontine veins. *5* Displaced interpeduncular veins

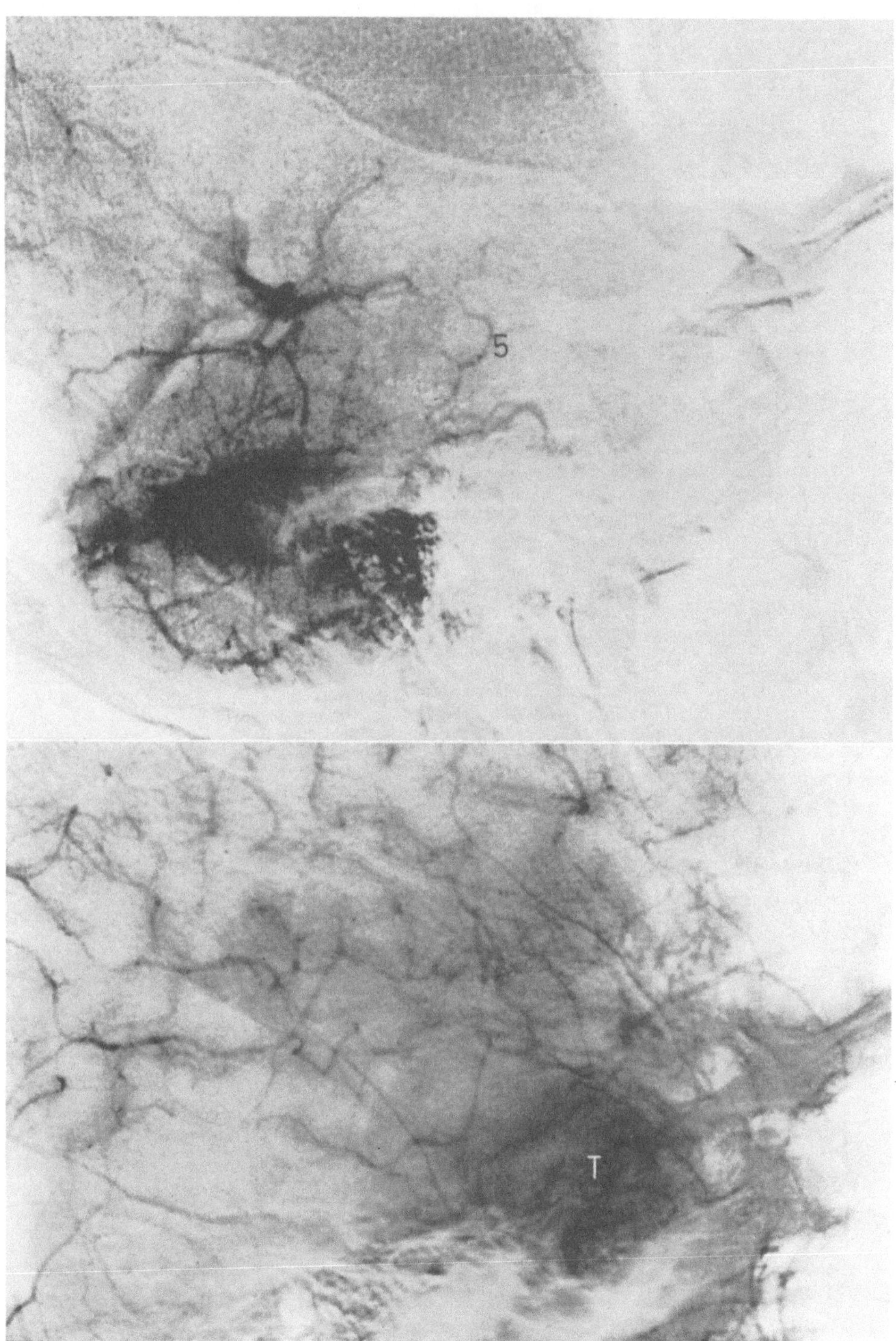

Fig. 119 b

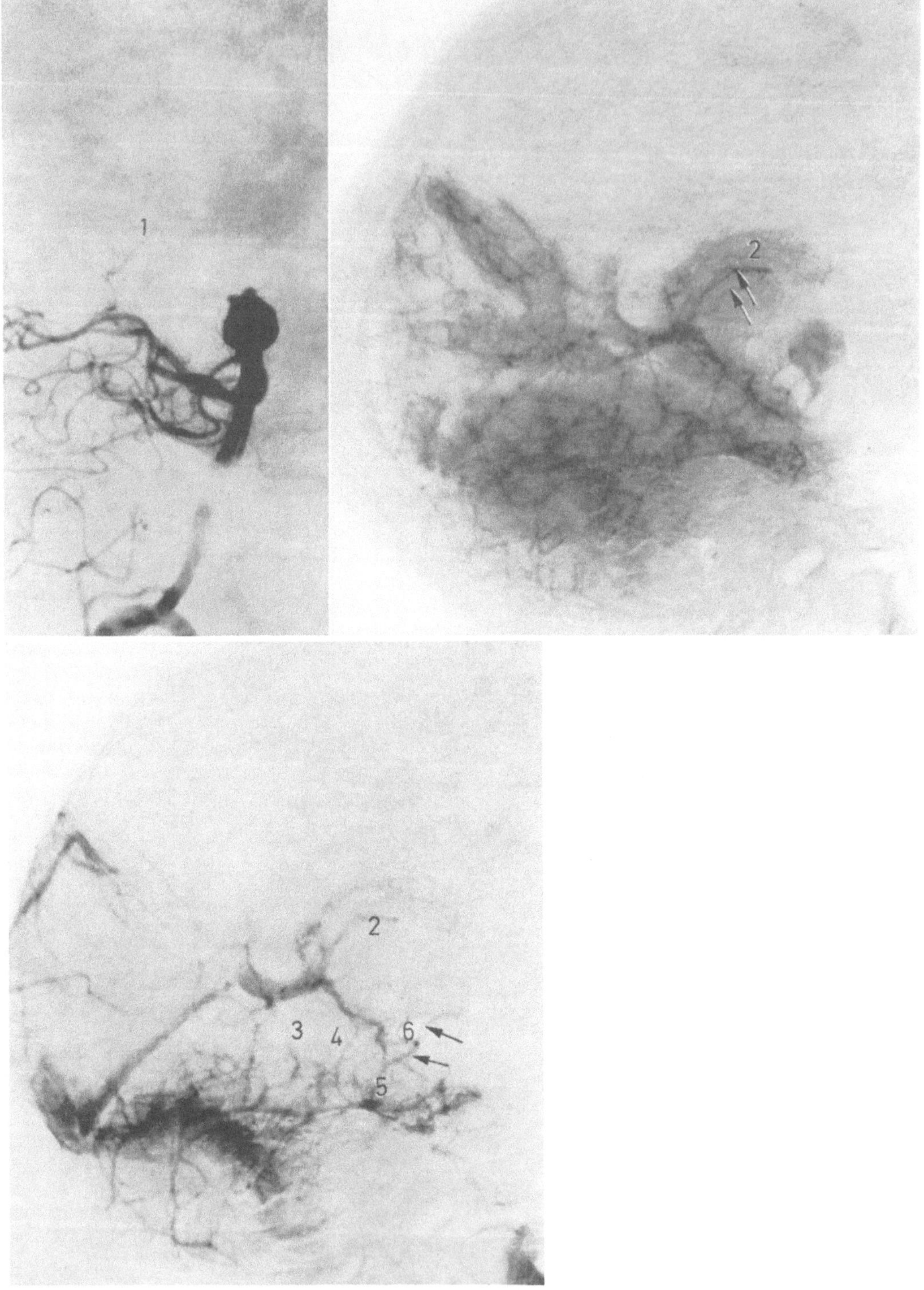

Fig. 120
Aneurysm of the superior extremity of the basilar trunk with enveloping hematoma. *1* Rigidity of the postero-medial choroidal artery. *2* Accentuation of the concavity of the thalamic veins. *3* Normal precentral vein. *4* Backward displacement of the lateral mesencephalic vein whose course is concave anteriorly. *5* Displaced prepontine veins. *6* Displaced interpeduncular veins

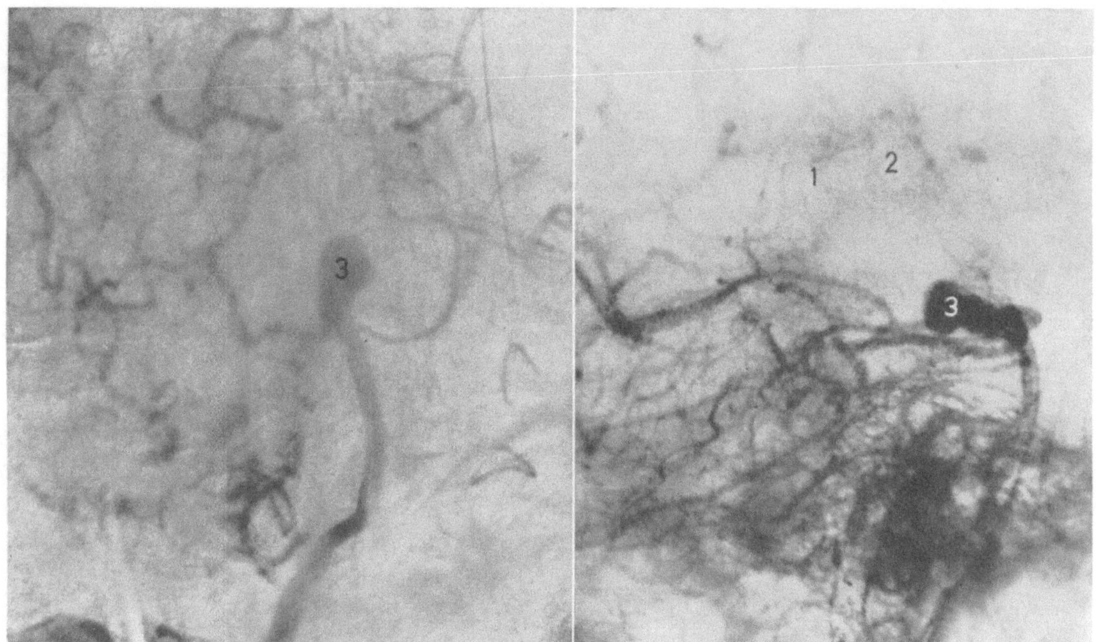

Fig. 121
Aneurysm of the superior extremity of the basilar trunk (*3*). Straightening of the postero-medial choroidal artery (*1*). Abnormal capillarography (*2*)

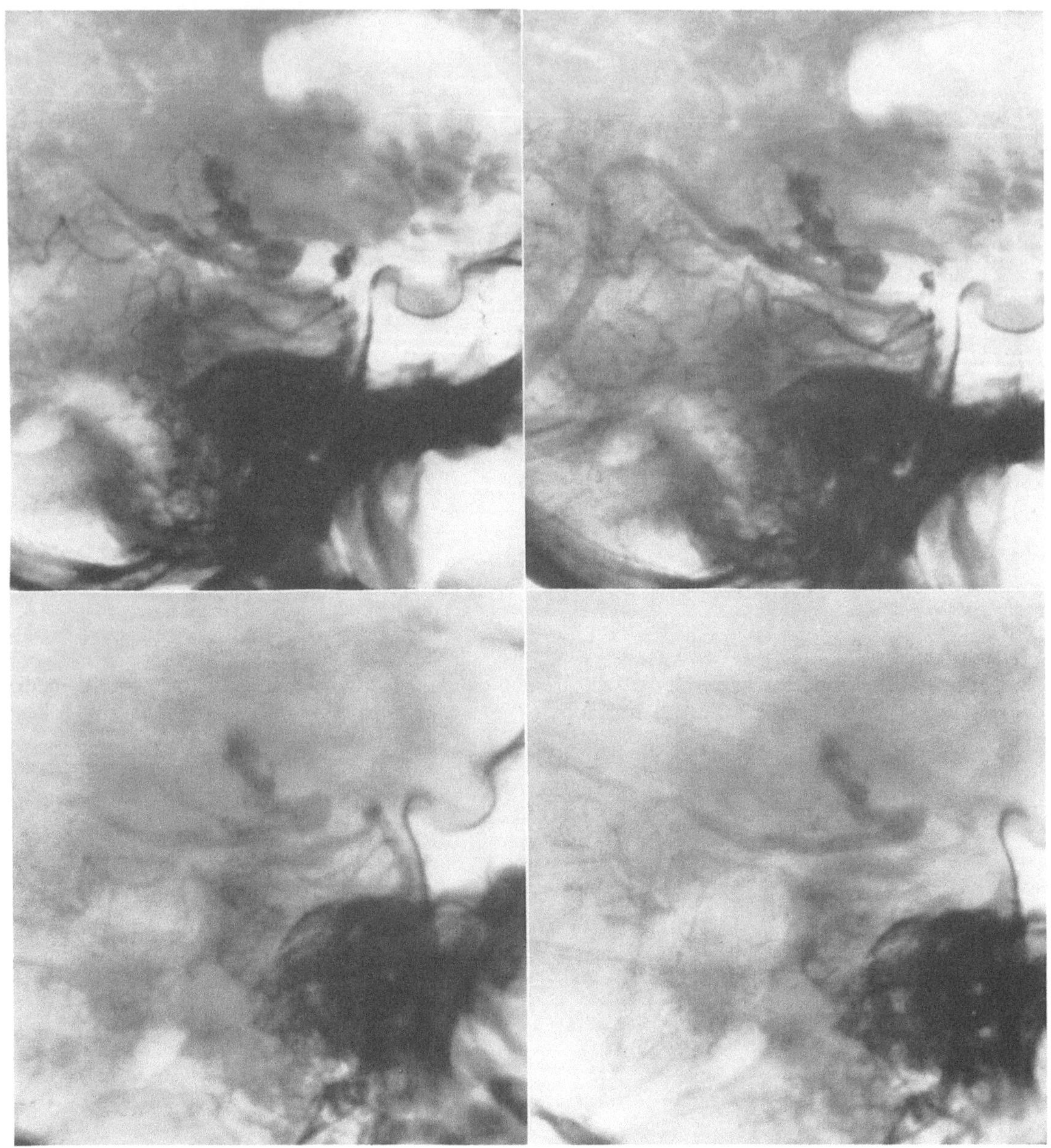

Fig. 122
Arteriovenous aneurysm formed by the colliculi quadrigemini et corporis geniculati arteries. Early venous drainage towards the straight sinus

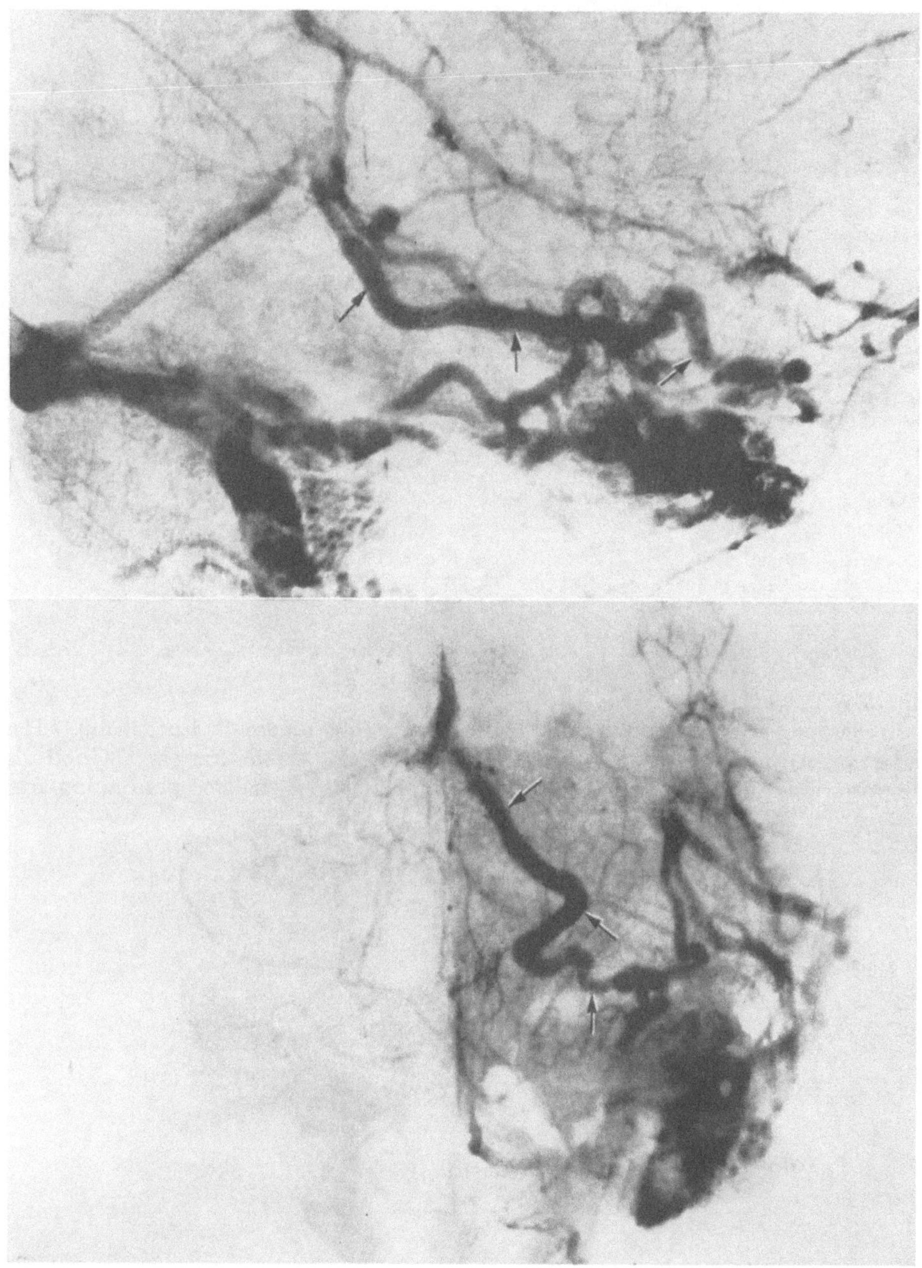

Fig. 123
Temporal arteriovenous aneurysm. Important dilatation of the basal vein draining an arteriovenous aneurysm. The normal collaterals of this hypertrophied vein are not visible

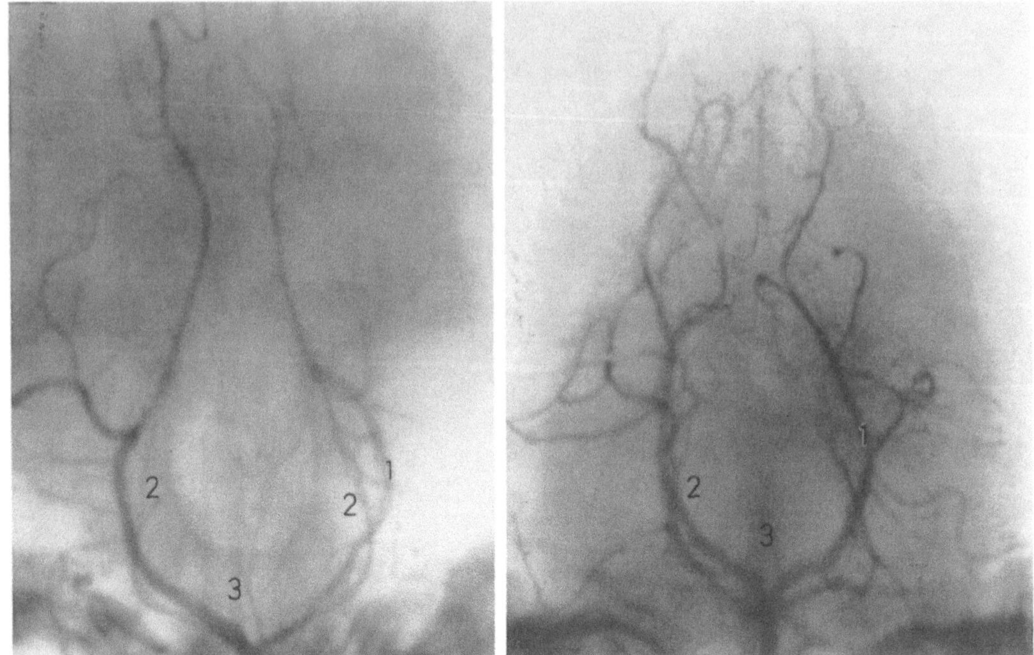

Fig. 124
Two examples of active non tumoral hydrocephaly (obstructive hydrocephaly). *1* Harmonious and symmetrical increase of curvature of the posterior cerebral artery. *2* Good visibility of the posterior choroidal arteries. *3* Rigidity of the posterior thalamo-perforating arteries

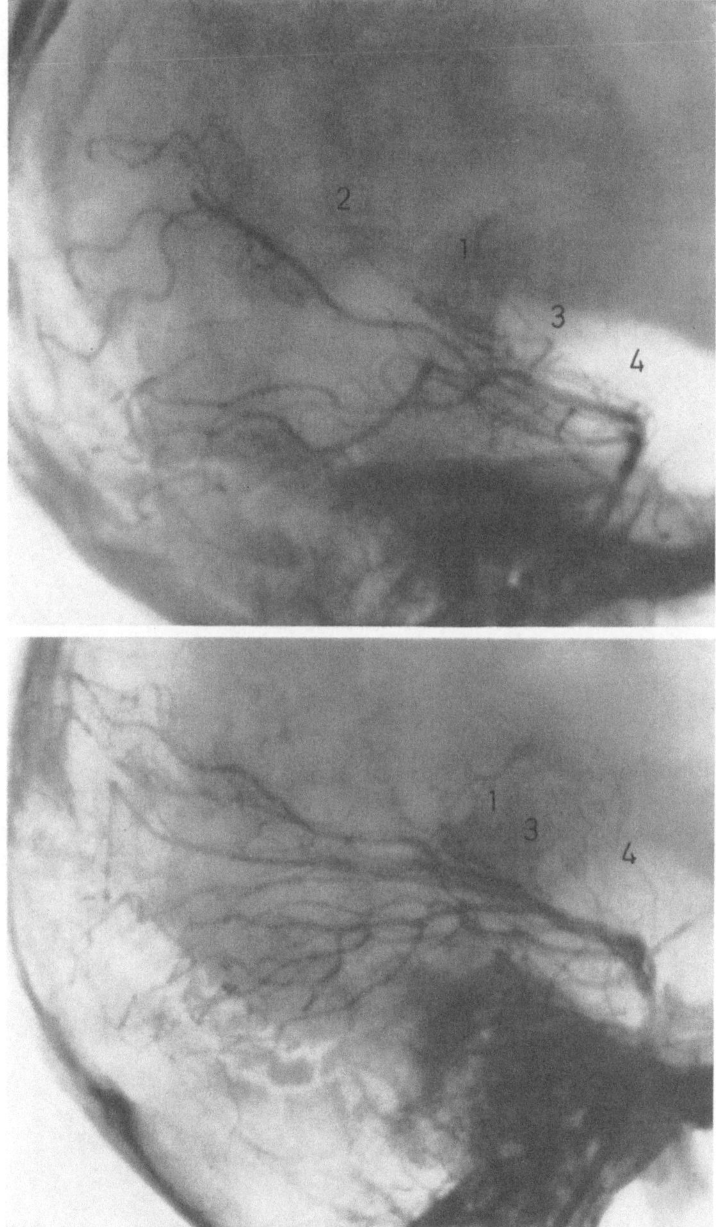

Fig. 125
Lateral projection of the arteries in cases of Fig. 124. *1* Crossing of the postero-medial and lateral choroidal arteries. *2* Good visibility of the hydrocephalic increase of curvature of the posterior pericallosal artery. *3* Good visibility of the colliculi quadrigemini et corporis geniculati arteries. *4* Good visibility of the thalamo-perforating arteries

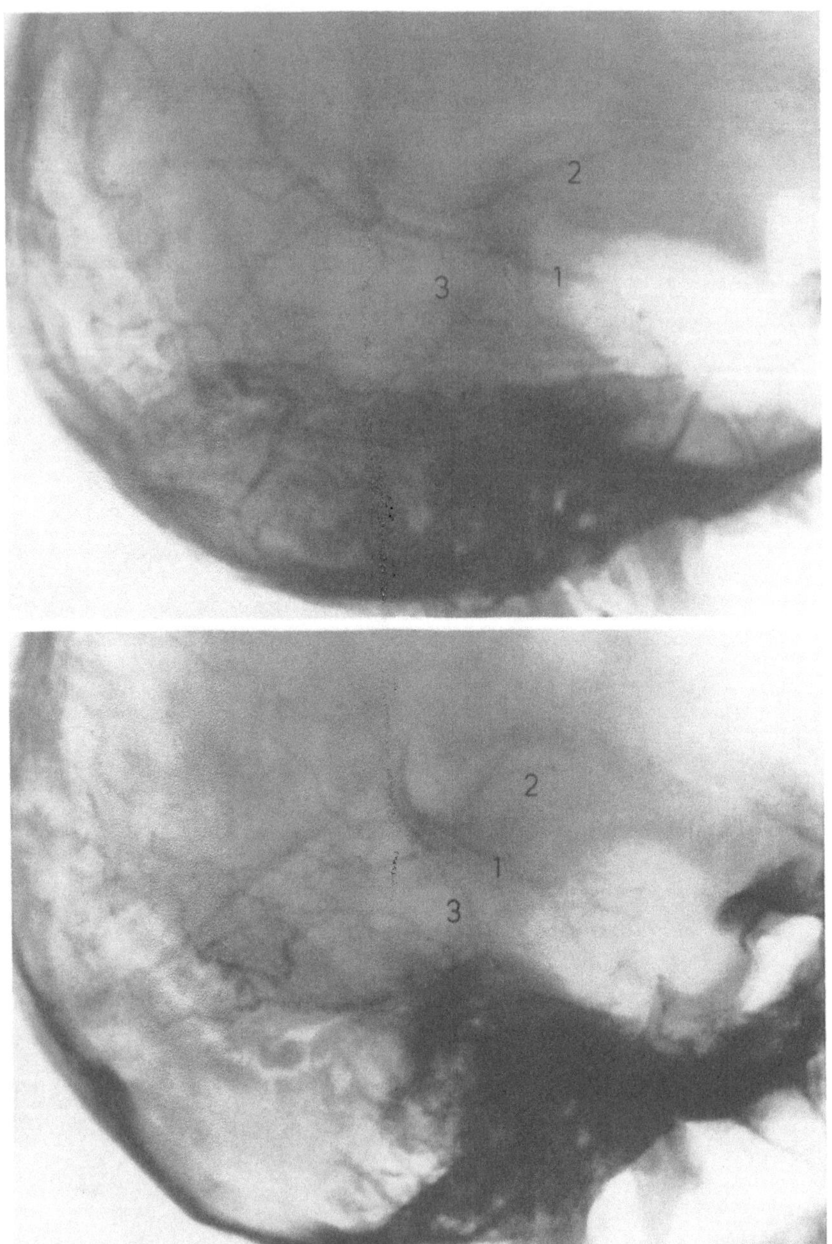

Fig. 126
Phlebography in cases of Figs. 124 and 125. *1* Flattening of the basal vein.
2 Dilatation of the superior thalamic vein. *3* Normal lateral mesencephalic
vein in one case (above); this vein is displaced towards the front in the
other case (below)

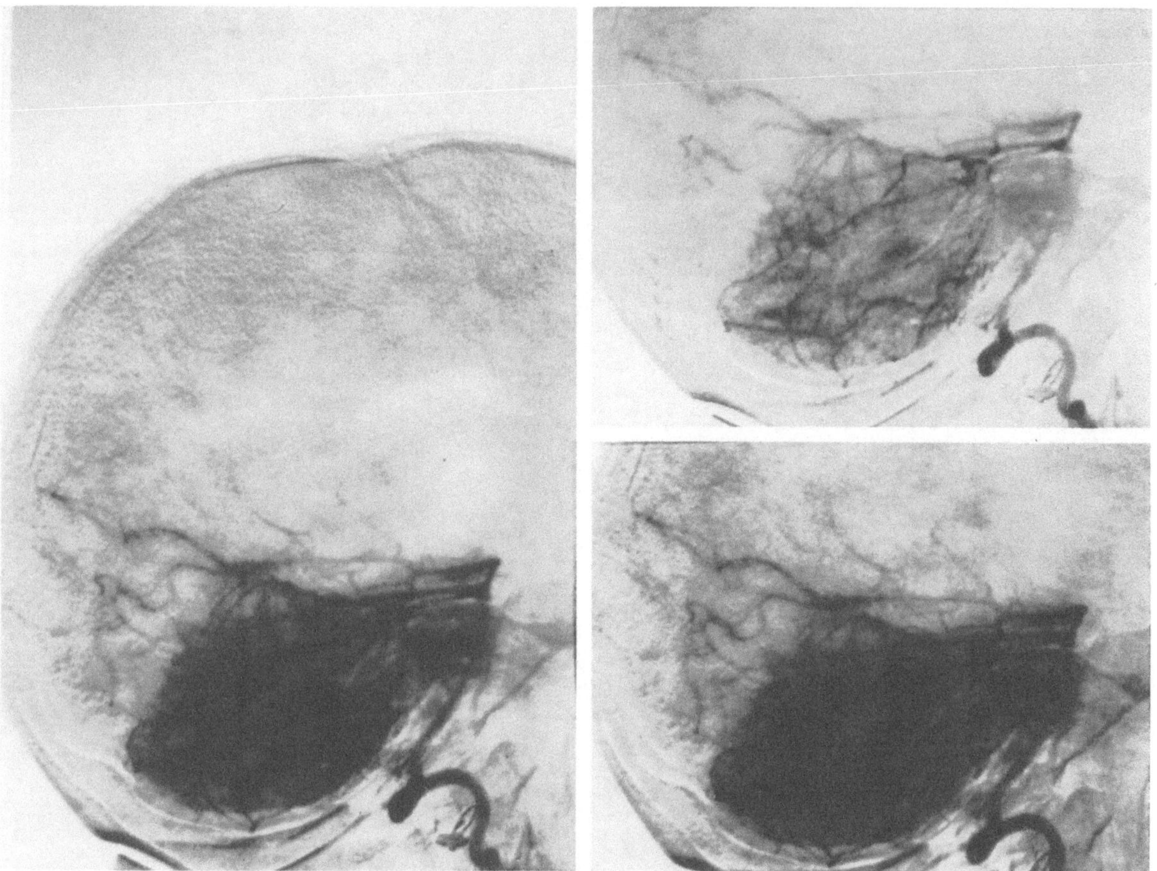

Fig. 127
Very dense capillarography in the entire posterior fossa due to vascular stasis. Intracranial hypertension due to tumour of the mesencephalic region

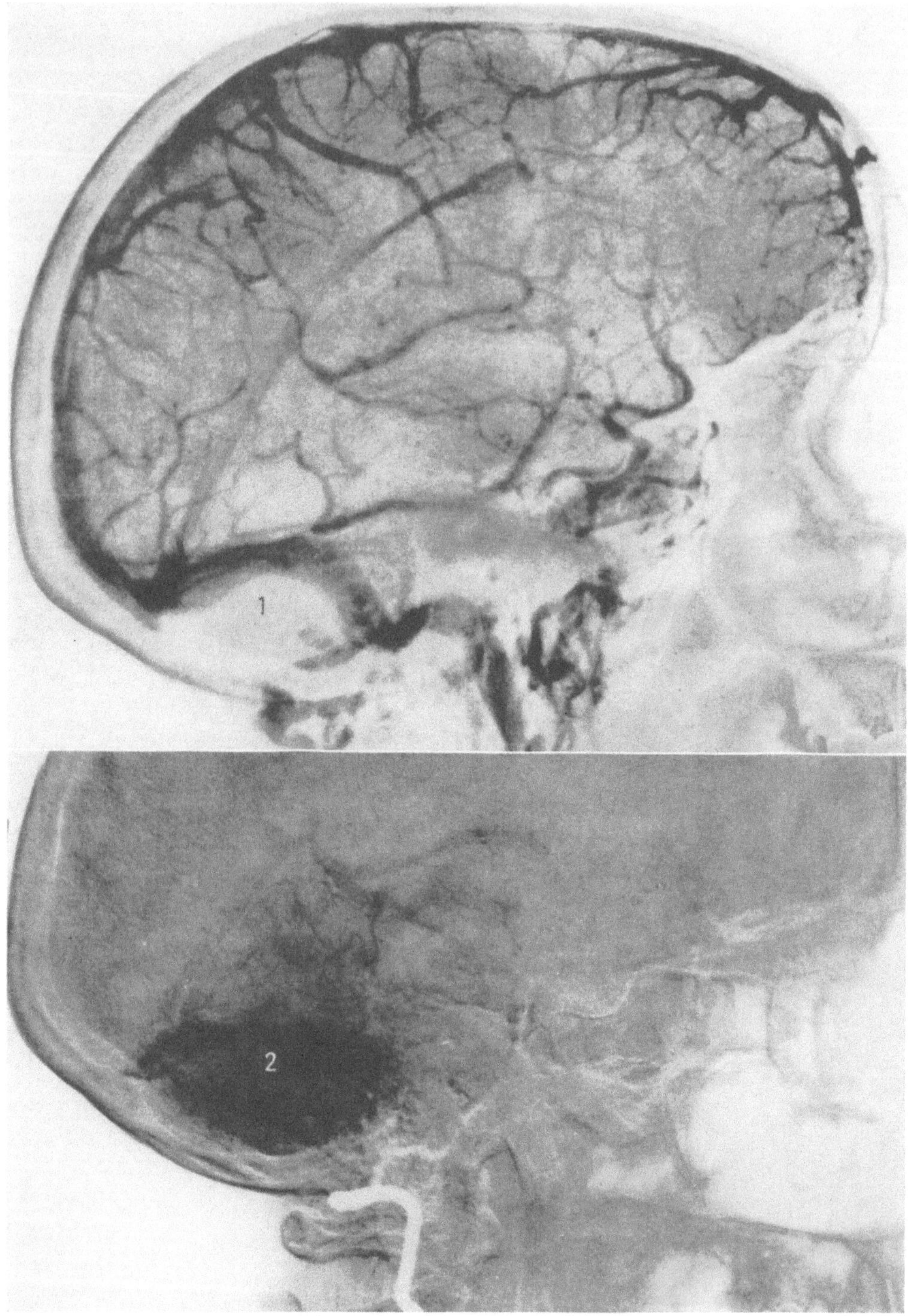

Fig. 128a
Tumour in the mesencephalic area (see also Fig. 106). Top: Carotid angiography. There is no contrast medium in the infratentorial space (*1*). Bottom: Vertebral angiography. The infratentorial space appears highly contrasted due to the capillary stasis (*2*)

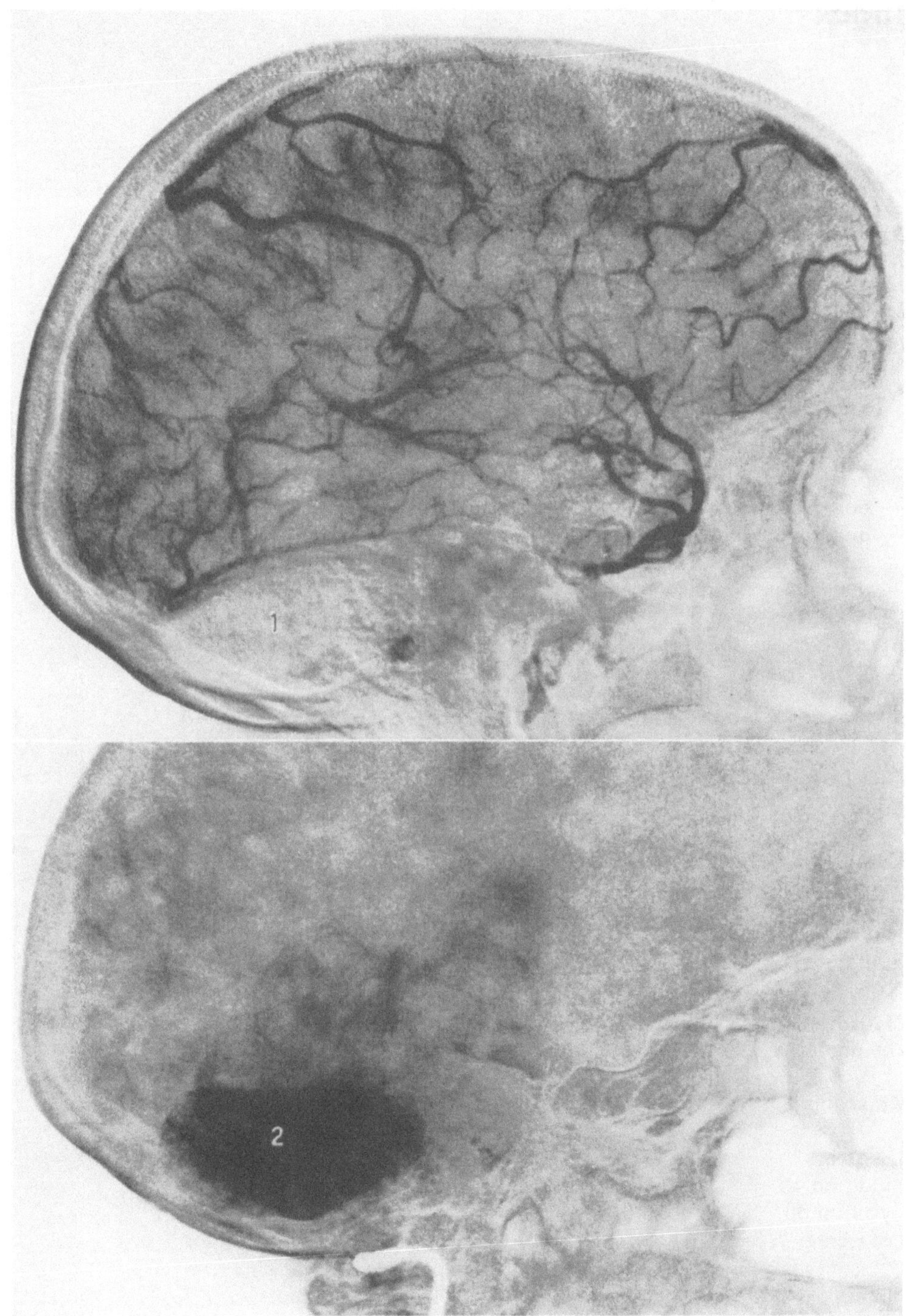

Fig. 128b